AF904683

SEPSIS

Edited by **Vijay Kumar**

Sepsis
http://dx.doi.org/10.5772/65611
Edited by Vijay Kumar

Contributors

Yukio Imamura, Yuki Murakami, Naoya Matsumoto, Hisatake Matsumoto, Kentaro Shimizu, Hiroshi Ogura, Takeshi Shimazu, Takashi Jin, Satoko Mitani, Natalia Beloborodova, Julie Chao, Vasilios Papaioannou, Alice Vassiliou, Stylianos E. Orfanos, Anastasia Kotanidou, Wiwat Chancharoenthana, Asada Leelahavanichkul, Somchai Eiam-Ong, Fabiano Pinheiro Da Silva, Mike Hamasaki, Marcel Machado

Published by InTech
Janeza Trdine 9, 51000 Rijeka, Croatia

© The Editor(s) and the Author(s) 2017
The moral rights of the editor(s) and the author(s) have been asserted.
All rights to the book as a whole are reserved by InTech. The book as a whole (compilation) cannot be reproduced, distributed or used for commercial or non-commercial purposes without InTech's written permission. Enquiries concerning the use of the book should be directed to InTech's rights and permissions department (permissions@intechopen.com).
Violations are liable to prosecution under the governing Copyright Law.

CC BY

Individual chapters of this publication are distributed under the terms of the Creative Commons Attribution 3.0 Unported License which permits commercial use, distribution and reproduction of the individual chapters, provided the original author(s) and source publication are appropriately acknowledged. More details and guidelines concerning content reuse and adaptation can be found at http://www.intechopen.com/copyright-policy.html.

Notice

Statements and opinions expressed in the chapters are these of the individual contributors and not necessarily those of the editors or publisher. No responsibility is accepted for the accuracy of information contained in the published chapters. The publisher assumes no responsibility for any damage or injury to persons or property arising out of the use of any materials, instructions, methods or ideas contained in the book.

Publishing Process Manager Nina Kalinic
Technical Editor SPi Global
Cover InTech Design team

First published August, 2017
Printed in Croatia
Legal deposit, Croatia: National and University Library in Zagreb

Additional hard copies can be obtained from orders@intechopen.com

Sepsis, Edited by Vijay Kumar
p. cm.
Print ISBN 978-953-51-3395-7
Online ISBN 978-953-51-3396-4

We are IntechOpen, the world's leading publisher of Open Access books

Built by scientists, for scientists

3,650+
Open access books available

114,000+
International authors and editors

118M+
Downloads

151
Countries delivered to

Our authors are among the
Top 1%
most cited scientists

12.2%
Contributors from top 500 universities

WEB OF SCIENCE™

Selection of our books indexed in the Book Citation Index in Web of Science™ Core Collection (BKCI)

Interested in publishing with us?
Contact book.department@intechopen.com

Numbers displayed above are based on latest data collected.
For more information visit www.intechopen.com

For EU product safety concerns:
IN TECH d.o.o., Prolaz Marije Krucifikse Kozulić 3, 51000 Rijeka, Croatia,
info@intechopen.com or visit our website at intechopen.com.

Meet the editor

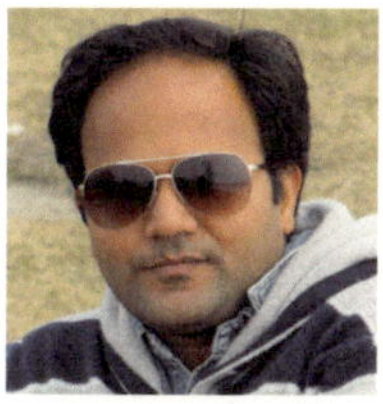

Dr. Kumar has more than 13 years of research experience in the field of bacterial sepsis along with other acute bacterial infections (i.e., pneumonia), innate immunity, and inflammation. He completed his PhD degree in June 2009 from the Department of Microbiology, Panjab University, Chandigarh, India. Thereafter, he moved internationally and worked as a postdoctoral researcher at various hospitals and universities in Canada, that is, Sainte-Justine Hospital, University de Montreal, Montreal, Quebec (2009–2010); Queens's University, Kingston, ON (2010–2012); and Sunnybrook Health Science Centre, University of Toronto, Toronto, ON (2012–2013). He worked with Translational Immunology Group at Trinity College, Dublin, Ireland (2014–2015). Currently, he is working with Children Health Clinical Unit, Faculty of Medicine at University of Queensland, Brisbane, Queensland, Australia. Dr. Kumar is the recipient of the prestigious "Piero Periti Review Article Award" for the year 2008, awarded by the *Journal of Chemotherapy* in the field of immunomodulation and antimicrobials for the article entitled "Innate Immunity in Sepsis Pathogenesis and Its Modulation: New Immunomodulatory Targets Revealed." He is the recipient of junior research and senior research fellowship [JRF and SRF (2004–2009)] offered by the Indian Council of Medical Research (ICMR), New Delhi, India. He has been awarded 13 travel awards to attend various international conferences in the field of sepsis and immunity. Till now, he has published 40 publications in peer-reviewed international journals in this field. He is also serving as an invited reviewer for many international journals.

Contents

Preface

Sepsis is a quintessential medical problem for physicians, intensive care unit (ICU) specialist, as well as biomedical researchers including microbiologists, immunologists, and pharmacologists involved in care and management of patients with sepsis and development of techniques for its early diagnosis, pathogenesis, and potential therapeutic targets. Study of sepsis in itself leads to the development of a different branch of medicine/medical sciences, as it can be seen in a wide variety of hosts from neonates to old-age population. Also, it can originate from different causes of the infection that is Gram-negative and Gram-positive bacteria, viruses, fungi, and parasites. Additionally, like other branches of science, the field of sepsis has also kept changing, for example, as per the Third International Consensus Definitions for Sepsis and Septic Shock (Sepsis-3) in 2016, the term systemic inflammatory response syndrome (SIRS) has been omitted from sepsis, and the term sepsis is now defined as life-threatening organ dysfunction caused by a dysregulated host response to infection systemically. Additionally, for clinical operationalization, Sequential [sepsis-related] Organ Failure Assessment (SOFA) score has now been introduced in 2016. Thus, this book is designed to keep its readers up to date in the continuously developing field of sepsis. Each section will prove helpful to students and researchers interested in the field of sepsis research. I hope this first edition of the book entitled *Sepsis* will convey its dynamism to its readers with chapters including metabolic interaction between pathogen and host during sepsis pathogenesis, age dependency in sepsis in pathogenesis, acute kidney injury in sepsis, and kallistatin-mediated immunoregulatory mechanism during sepsis along with developments in early diagnostic techniques for sepsis and sepsis-associated encephalitis. The field of sepsis research is continuously developing and changing very fast with the scientific advancement. Each chapter is written by an expert in the field, but, in some areas, there may be differences of opinion expressed by equally established authors. I will ask the readers to take this in note and follow the development and advancement in the sepsis research on both clinical and basic science levels.

Vijay Kumar, PhD
Research Fellow
Children's Health Clinical Unit, Queensland
Faculty of Medicine
University of Queensland, Brisbane
Queensland, Australia

Section 1

Metabolic Interaction Between Pathogen and Host During Sepsis

Chapter 1

Interaction of Host-Microbial Metabolism in Sepsis

Beloborodova Natalia Vladimirovna

Additional information is available at the end of the chapter

http://dx.doi.org/10.5772/68046

Abstract

The majority of species of the human gut microbiota is not cultivated on artificial nutrient media, but they are included in the functioning of microbial metabolic conveyor. Between the numerous gut bacteria (transmitter) and billions of intracellular mitochondria (receiver), the function of signaling molecules performs aromatic metabolites. Sepsis destroys the coordinated work of the indigenous anaerobic microflora. This leads to the imbalance of aromatic microbial metabolites (AMM). We hypothesized and proved diagnostic and pathogenic significance of this. First, deficiency of the end products of microbial metabolism—lipophilic AMM (PhPA and derivatives-cinnamic and benzoic acids) in sepsis, and second, excessive accumulation in blood of intermediate products named, "sepsis-associated" AMM—both lead to the development of mitochondrial dysfunction. Particularly, the total suppressed production of mROS can manifest by "hibernate-like state" of cells and lead to MOF. The participation of aromatic metabolites in the development of septic shock can be explained by the inhibition of tyrosine hydroxylase and impaired synthesis of catecholamines. In clinical research, the high levels of "sepsis-associated" AMM (p-HPhAA, p-HPhLA, and PhLA) correlate with the severity according to APACHE II, Sepsis-related Organ Failure Assessments (SOFA) score and mortality. To improve the survival of ICU patients, requires more attention to the role of imbalance of microbial metabolites in sepsis.

Keywords: sepsis, microbiota, aromatic microbial metabolites, organ dysfunction, mitochondrial dysfunction, tyrosine, septic shock

1. Introduction

Currently, improvement of diagnostic and medical technologies in surgery and intensive care allows us to provide real treatment of patients, including previously considered incurable. However, the development of infectious complications, syndrome of multiple organ failure (MOF), and septic shock significantly worsens the results. Every year the problem of

INTECH
open science | open minds

© 2017 The Author(s). Licensee InTech. This chapter is distributed under the terms of the Creative Commons Attribution License (http://creativecommons.org/licenses/by/3.0), which permits unrestricted use, distribution, and reproduction in any medium, provided the original work is properly cited. (cc) BY

increasing sepsis-associated mortality becomes more acute in different categories of high-risk patients (e.g., premature infants and elderly, patients with cancer, diabetes mellitus, states after injuries, strokes, surgeries, transplants, etc.). Further progress in medicine is impossible without a revision of basic ideas about the important role of metabolic disturbances of the microbiota in the pathogenesis of sepsis. Nowadays, the question of the role of the microbiota comes to the forefront. Numerous research teams conduct in-depth study using the most contemporary technologies, including metagenomics sequencing, etc. Identifying the microbial DNA and RNA, scientists try to decipher hundreds of species of microorganisms living in the human gut. It is important to note that the majority of species of the intestinal microbiota of man is not cultivated on artificial nutrient media, but is included in the functioning of multistage microbial metabolic reactor [1]. More and more data appear on crosstalk between the organism and host microbial ecology, including epigenomic and metagenomic programming with the involvement of gut microbiota [2]. There are serious reasons to believe that in order to decipher mechanisms of sepsis, it is essential to evaluate the functional component of the microbial metabolism. Integration of the metabolism of the host and its normal microbiota provides the human health sepsis means a profound failure in the general metabolic pathways of man and microbiota, often irreversible that leads to unfavorable outcome.

The absence of a unique approach to an objective assessment of vital threat of damage in the main integration points of host-microbial metabolism makes difficult an early diagnosis, prognosis, and targeted treatment of sepsis. In this chapter, we summarize knowledge available from the literature and the results of our own experience of research, the pathogenetic significance of some microbial metabolites in sepsis—at the organismal, cellular, and subcellular levels.

2. Microbial metabolism in healthy and in sepsis

The symbiosis of the host and its microbiota exists due to the large number and variety of species of bacteria (aerobic, facultative anaerobic, and strict anaerobic bacteria). The microecological system is the boundary of the inner sterile environment from the external world (all of the mucous membranes and skin), but most richly represented in the gut microbiota.

A large number of different types of microorganisms perform the biochemical functions as a multilevel "conveyor", which involved numerous members of the microbiota. The result depends on many factors. The quality and quantity of substrate (food components), the function of the stomach, pancreas, liver, gallbladder, and bowel motility, etc. definitely influence the metabolism of microbiota. At the same time, the diversity of species with different biochemical activity provides coordinated work of the microbiota. Therefore, in normal biotransformation of any of the substrates in the intestinal lumen takes place sequentially and ends with the formation of the final metabolites.

It is important to note that many microbial metabolites have biological activity and perform important functions in the host organism. They are necessary for the normal functioning of organs and systems. For example, fecal short-chain fatty acids (SCFAs) are important energy substrate for enterocytes. They provide functioning of the local immunological barrier, preventing bacterial translocation. SCFAs are sent directly into the cells of the intestinal epithelium and "delayed" at the level of the mucosa, therefore, normally they are not detected in the blood of healthy people. Other products of microbial metabolism permanently enter the internal environment of the organism (blood and lymph); therefore, they are called extracellular microbial metabolites or exometabolites.

In the body of a healthy person have well-functioning mechanisms to maintain the homeostasis of microbial metabolites at a constant level [3]. If microbial exometabolites enter the blood in excess amounts, they are neutralized in the liver (for example, phenol is converted into cresol), form sulfates and conjugates with amino acids (glycine and glutamine) and glucuronic acid, etc., then in the form of water-soluble compounds excreted in the urine.

MS-based metabolomics studies (using LC- and GH-MS) on germ-free (gnotobiotic) mammals showed that many classes of low molecular weight compounds (free or conjugate) in blood are of microbial origin [4]. For example, many phenolic metabolites, such as phenyl sulfate, p-kresol sulfate, conjugate of phenyl propionic, and cinnamic acids (phenylpropionylglicine and cinnamoylglicine) observed only in normal (conventional) animals. Concentrations of other phenolic compounds were many times higher in the blood of normal animals compared to germ-free animals, *p*-value 10^{-8} to 10^{-9}, such as phenyl benzoic conjugate (hippuric) and phenyl acetic conjugate (phenylacetylglycine).

The humans carry out their activities in close contact with the inhabiting microflora from the first day after birth to the last, i.e., throughout life. In ontogenesis, there created a system of human-microbiota, thanks to close and mutually beneficial metabolic integration [5]. The presence of integration of host-microbial metabolism is confirmed by the fact that

- the number of microbial cells inhabiting the human community is huge, according to some authors exceeds [6] or at least comparable [7] with the number of cells in the human body;
- high speed reproduction of microorganisms and cell renewal of the microbial community indicates active metabolic process in bacteria;
- qualitative and quantitative composition of biological community indicates the existence of mechanisms of regulation within the microbial community, the so-called "quorum sensing;"
- number of mechanisms of immunoreactivity aimed at maintaining a symbiotic relationship that indicates the existence of mutual regulation through a system of common metabolites and/or signaling molecules.

The results of our research allow us to assert that the number of products of microbial metabolism namely phenolic acids entering the bloodstream of critically ill patients in large amounts can block the respiratory chain of mitochondria, disrupting the functions of organs and tissues that are directly involved in the genesis of multiple organ failure (MOF).

These relationships change radically in patients with severe illnesses, reaching a maximum deviation from the norm in critical conditions, until the development of irreversible disorders of homeostasis and death of the host organisms. Massive tissue damage of any origin is accompanied by hypoxia, shortage of energetically plastic materials, which reflects violations of the metabolic processes of microorganism and influences the metabolism of its microbiota. When the host organism is under extreme conditions (massive hemorrhage, hypoxia, hypo- or hyperthermia, starvation, hypovolemia, poisoning, irradiation, etc.), that means the rapid changes in the environment of microorganisms inhabiting gut of host.

Sepsis is characterized by sudden depletion and simplification of the microbiota as follows:

- first of all, destroyed biofilms of microbial symbionts, namely indigenous anaerobes (*Bifidobacteria, Lactobacilli*, etc.) [8];
- facultative anaerobes (enterobacteria, staphylococci, etc.) form biofilms in the upper digestive tract (bacterial expansion in the small intestine) [9, 10];
- clinically it is manifested by the failure of intestinal barrier and bacterial translocation [11, 12];
- the blood circulating bacteria from gut "in search of" more favorable conditions, which are recorded as "bacteremia" [13];
- resistant to the ongoing antibiotic treatment, bacteria remains in the micro thrombus, exudate, and damaged epithelium/endothelium, forming local foci of infection [14].

3. Why aromatic microbial metabolites (AMM) are the most important in sepsis?

To study the metabolomics profile of biological fluids different technologies including the most gas chromatography-mass spectrometry (GC-MS), liquid chromatography-mass spectrometry (with two mass analyzers in one mass spec instrument) (LC-MS/MS), 1H (H)- (proton nuclear magnetic resonance) spectroscopy (NMR), etc. are used. Global metabolic profiling—spanning hundreds of small molecules—holds the potential to reveal not only host and microbial metabolites, novel biomarkers, but also provides insight into disease pathogenesis.

In our experiments, we used GC-MS analysis of blood serum, as in sepsis in the blood enters the microbial exometabolites from the intestine and from foci of infection. Blood microbial metabolites spread throughout the body to the cells of all organs (**Figure 1**). Comparing qualitative and quantitative composition of low molecular metabolites in the blood of different groups of patients, we found that most of qualitative and quantitative significant differences between the healthy and the sick are observed among aromatic metabolites. In the blood of healthy and sick people, we have identified and measured tens of aromatic metabolites such as phenol, benzole, and their derivatives (p-cresol, benzyl alcohol, benzoic acid, 2,4-dihydroxybenzoic acid, 3,4-dihydroxybenzoic acid, and p-hydroxybenzoic acid), carbolic acids (lactic, malic, fumaric, succinic, 2-ketoglutaric, 2-hydroxyglutaric, 2-hydroxybutyric, etc.), phenyl carboxylic acids (phenylacetic, p-hydroxyphenylacetic, 2-hydroxyphenylacetic, phenylpropionic, p-hydroxyphenyl propionic, cinnamic, p-hydroxyphenyl cinnamic, phenyllactic,

http://dx.doi.org/10.5772/68046

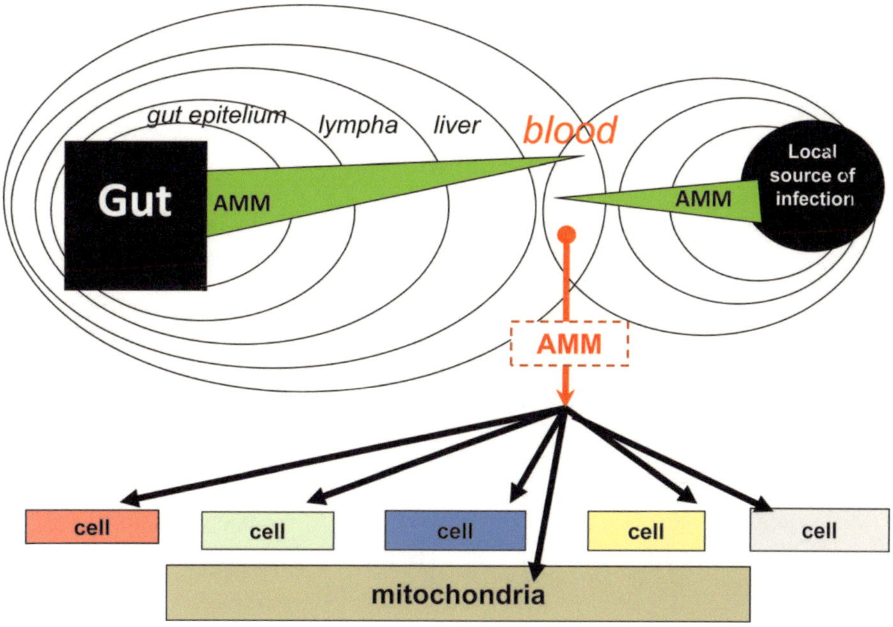

Figure 1. Sources and targets of serum aromatic microbial metabolites (AMM) in sepsis.

p-hydroxyphenyllactic, phenylpyruvic, p-hydroxyphenylpyruvic, and o-hydroxyphenylacetic), indolic acids (1-indoleacetic acid and 3-indoleacetic acid), etc.

It proved the microbial origin of phenyl carboxylic acids in the human body [15]. The examination and comparison of different groups of people discovered that some aromatic metabolites in the blood of patients with sepsis strongly differed from all other groups of patients. We named these compounds as "sepsis-associated" aromatic microbial metabolites (AMM). On chemical structure, they can be attributed to phenolic or phenyl carboxylic acids (**Figure 2**).

Jenner et al. [16] analyzed the profile of aromatic compounds (about 50) in the gut of healthy people. The results showed that they are quantitatively dominated by such metabolites

$$\text{PhAA} > \text{p-HPhAA} > 3,4\ \text{di-HCinA} > \text{PhPA} > \text{BA} \tag{1}$$

Our research has shown that most of these AMMs are also present in the serum of healthy people [17], but in a different ratio:

$$\text{p-HPhLA} > \text{BA} > \text{p-HPhAA} > \text{PhAA} > \text{PhLA} > \text{PhPA} \tag{2}$$

Differences in the proportion of AMM in the blood compared to the intestine can be explained by the fact that most hydrophilic (p-HPhAA, p-HPhLA, and PhLA) metabolites are excreted by the kidneys, while lipophilic metabolites (BA, PhAA, and PhPA) are absorbed by cells of tissue barriers (intestinal wall, lymphoid tissue, liver, vascular endothelium, etc.).

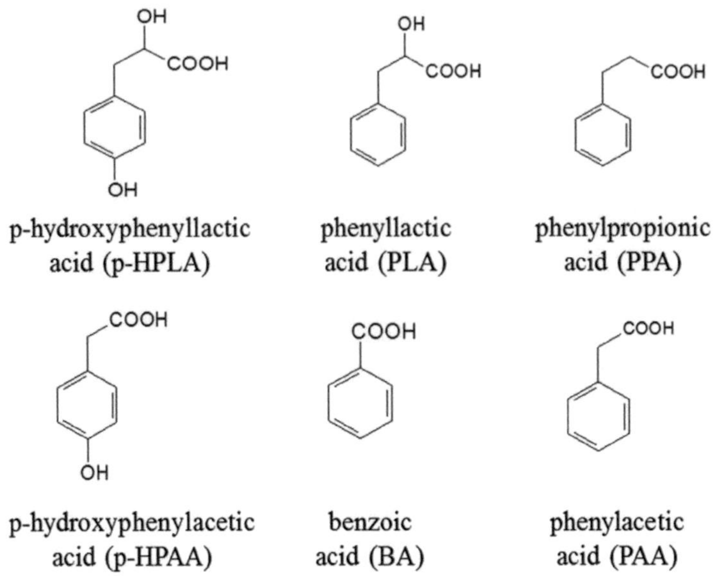

Figure 2. "Sepsis-associated" aromatic microbial metabolites (AMM).

It is important to note that all patients with a diagnosis of sepsis discovered the highest levels in the serum of PhLA, p-HPhLA, p-HPhAA, and always-no PhPA [18].

The comparisons of the levels of microbial aromatic metabolites (AMM) in the blood of septic patients versus a normal level of metabolites in the blood and in bowel (fecal water) of healthy are presented in **Table 1**.

Figure 3 presents visual comparison data on serum concentrations of six AMM (GC-MS, ng/ml) in groups of healthy and patients with chronic heart failure, familial mediterranean fever (FMF), pneumonia, and sepsis. It is important to note that the concentration of lipophilic AMM is so small that the image is almost not visible. At the same time, the concentration of the three "sepsis-associated acids" (PhLA, p-HPhLA, and p-HPhAA) in patients with sepsis greatly exceeds the levels of AMM when comparing groups.

The studies had different questions as follows:

1. Does not such a high level of AMM in violation of their elimination from the body, for example, in renal or hepatic failure (excluding sepsis)?
2. Increase of sepsis-associated AMM in patients with severe trauma without sepsis?
3. What about patients with phenylketonuria?

After the examination of six different groups of patients, such doubts were dispelled and again shows that sepsis is characterized by increase of all three "sepsis-associated" AMM—PhLA, p-HPhLA, and p-HPhAA (**Figure 4**).

AMM	AMM in the blood of septic patients, μM, median (IR 25–75%)	AMM in the blood of healthy, μM, median (IR 25–75%)	AMM in the bowel (faecal water) of healthy, data from [7], μM
Lipophilic AMM			
PhPA	*nd**	0,2 (0,1–0,4)	200-600
PhAA	0,4 (0,1–0,7)	0,4 (0,3–0,6)	400-1100
BA	0,9 (0,8–2,0)	0,7 (0,6–0,8)	23-25
Hydrophilic AMM			
di-HCinA	*nd*	*nd*	50-200
PhLA	2,7 (1,4–5,1)	0,3 (0,2–0,4)	*nd*
p-HPhLA	7,6 (2,9–15,5)	1,1 (0,9–2,0)	*nd*
p-HPhAA	14,1 (7,8–35,9)	0,5 (0,4–0,6)	60-400

* *nd*, not detected.

Table 1. The levels of microbial aromatic metabolites (AMM) in the blood of septic patients versus a normal level of metabolites in the blood and in bowel (faecal water) of healthy.

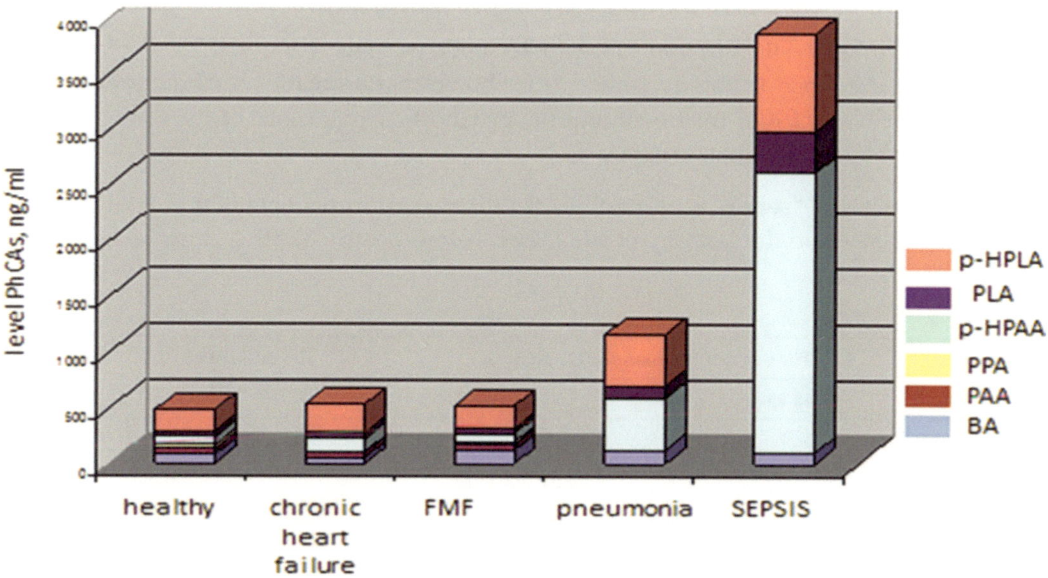

Figure 3. High serum concentrations of p-HPhAA, p-HPhLA, and PhLA (GC/MS, ng/ml) in septic patients versus healthy and chronic heart failure, familial mediterranean fever (FMF), and pneumonia.

The first report on the potential diagnostic value of the level of AMM in sepsis has been reported to us on the International Sepsis Forum (ISF-2007, Paris) and then was published [19]. There was a presentation on the results of GC-MS analysis, which revealed the highest

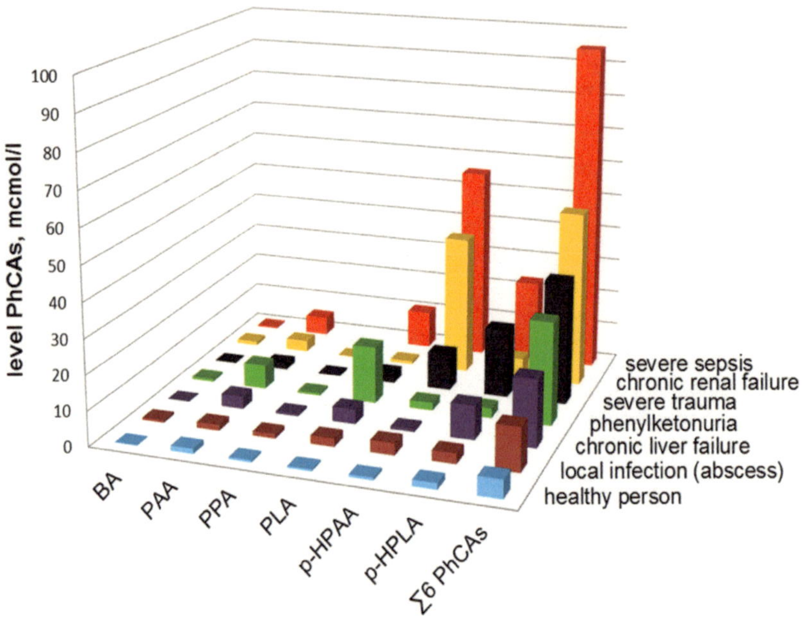

Figure 4. The levels of six phenyl carboxylic acids in blood of six groups of patients (GC-MS, μM).

levels of p-HPhAA, p-HPhLA, and PhLA in 44 septic patients. Then, the levels of AMM in patients were examined in the dynamics. It is shown that aromatic metabolites accurately reflect the efficiency of ICU treatment and the prognostic significance of the some aromatic metabolites is higher than that of lactate [20].

The highest levels of "sepsis-associated" AMM discovered in patients with a fatal outcome in end-stage sepsis, on the last day of life (<24 h before death). **Table 2** shows a significant

Parameter	Time to death (retrospective analysis)		The multiplicity of changes, Me	*p*=
	48-25 h	24-0 h		
MODS_2	5 (3—7)	9 (6—10)	1,8	<0.001
Lactate, μM	3,6 (2,4—5,1)	4,2 (3,0—10,6)	1,2	0.030
PhLA, μM, median (IR 25-75%)	4,27 (2,14—9,33)	7,97 (5,07—17,90)	1,9	<0.001
p-HPhAA, μM, median (IR 25-75%)	10,45 (1,99—25,81)	20,14 (7,27—65,49)	1,9	<0.001
p-HPhLA, μM, median (IR 25-75%)	9,14 (5,73—25,51)	22,06 (13,64—67,04)	2,4	<0.001
∑3 AMM, μM, median (IR 25-75%)	33,47 (12,40—63,98)	78,02 (38,92—156,26)	2,3	<0.001

Table 2. Some clinical and laboratory data of the monitoring terminal ICU patients in the last 2 days of life (n = 34).

increase in the level of AMM (p-HPhAA, p-HPhLA, and PhLA) in the last 2 days of life in terminal ICU patients (n-34) and significantly the highest concentration for the moment of death.

Later, the relationship was also found between p-HPhLA and 28-day mortality in a large study from Roger et al., after analysis of metabolic profiling of plasma samples from 90 ICU subjects [21].

These facts point to the possible own biological activity of AMM and their direct participation in the mechanisms of pathogenesis and thanatogenesis of sepsis.

4. The role of microbial metabolites in the pathogenesis of sepsis

4.1. Bacterial load and neutrophils

Studies have confirmed that increased bacterial load is accompanied by an increase in the total blood concentration of AMM [22] that contributes to the transition from local infection to sepsis. This can be observed with late diagnosis, inadequate antibiotic therapy, or delayed surgical rehabilitation of the infection focus. So, when comparing patients with different severity of bacterial infection, it is shown that in the group of patients with sepsis, serum concentrations of hydrophilic AMM were significantly higher versus the group of local infections of skin and soft tissues [23].

It is shown that the AMM level reflects the severity of the infectious process and is directly correlated with the number of clinical signs of inflammation, indicators of severity APACHEII and SOFA scores [24].

Neutrophils are the first line of defense against bacteria. They quickly migrate to the site of infection or inflammation, neutralize foreign particles, phagocytose, and destroy bacteria. Polymorphonuclear leukocytes also transmit signals to other cells of the nonspecific immune system about the threat of invasion of foreign agents. Neutrophil dysfunction is one of the key mechanisms of severe infection and sepsis development.

Thus, the microbial load in sepsis associated with microbial metabolites. To test the hypothesis about the influence of AMM on the phagocytic activity of neutrophils, experiments were conducted *in vitro*. It was shown that *in vitro* some sepsis-associated AMM in clinically relevant concentrations are able to inhibit phagocytic activity of neutrophils. In experiments with neutrophils observed the disruption caused by the influence of AMM *in vitro*. They were associated with suppressed production of ROS and similar to those found in patients with sepsis; therefore, among the reasons for mitochondrial dysfunction in sepsis can play an important role in the imbalance of microbial metabolites [25].

4.2. Organ dysfunction

Retrospective analysis of the causes of deaths by group of authors (Vincent, Nelson, and Williams), using a database of 28 countries, which contains all information about 4459 patients with severe sepsis [26]. It has been shown that for the period, by the 28th day from the time of diagnosis of sepsis died 1201 patients and mortality was 27%. The analysis showed that all the deceased patients showed an increase in the dynamics of the severity of organ disorders, which were objectively evaluated by the growing points on the SOFA scale. The main causes of death were multiple organ failure (MOF) associated with sepsis (43%) and refractory septic shock (22.6%). At the same time, the results of histological findings in postmortem studies of organs and tissues from patients, who died from sepsis, are not consistent with the degree of the organ dysfunction. Cells of heart, kidney, liver, and lungs in the death of sepsis were subjected to minimal changes. In patients with clinical signs of myocardial depression had no data on the damage of cardiomyocytes. Kidney (nephrons and tubules) were intact. That is, the organs looked normal while they are clinically noted MOF with fatal outcome [27]. Thus, it is quite reasonable today in the center of attention—the causes and mechanisms of MOF in patients with sepsis [28].

Fortunately, more than half of patients with sepsis survive. Organ dysfunction in sepsis is sometimes called "hibernation-like state" from the point of view of its reversibility [29]. In other words, MOF means something disrupts normal functioning of the cells, in sepsis it is not so much hypoxia, but how much a reduction in energy availability. Unique to sepsis are the coexisting findings: metabolic acidosis means increased oxygen demand, at the same time recorded a decrease of oxygen consumption. The greatest attention is paid to study mitochondrial mechanisms of sepsis-induced organ failure.

It is known that the mitochondria in human cells are similar to bacteria not only in size. Mitochondria have their own DNA, which is similar to bacterial DNA and very different from the DNA of human cells. Mitochondria and bacteria have also some similar pathways for energy production. A number of other biological characteristics also point to a prokaryotic origin of mitochondria in ontogenesis [30].

4.3. Mitochondrial dysfunction

According to the authors, mitochondria reduce the supply of energy to the cell to cause metabolic shutdown. This adaptive mechanism is similar to hibernation, it prevents massive cell death and thereby, gives a chance of complete recovery of organ function after recovery in survivors [31].

The concept of mitochondrial dysfunction and bioenergetics failure during sepsis is not new [32], but it remains unclear why in sepsis does this unique mechanism and what role bacteria play. Our experimental approaches have revealed the influence of AMM on mitochondrial function that have novel and interesting findings [33]. It turned out that some aromatic microbial metabolites are able to inhibit the NAD-dependent mitochondrial respiration. It is shown that the degree of inhibition depends on the chemical structure of metabolites [34]. In the experiment, *in vitro* the degree of inhibition of respiration of mitochondria by cinnamic acid was taken as 100% (**Figure 5**). We can conclude that inhibition of mitochondrial respiration can only occupy lipophilic AMM and its derivates (benzoic and cinnamic acids are metabolites of PhPA).

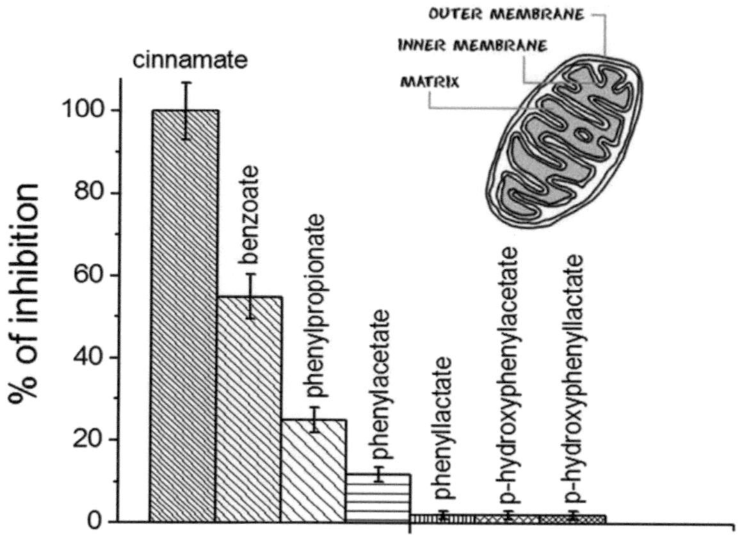

The inhibition of NAD-dependent respiration of mitochondria by cinnamic acid was taken to be 100%. The concentration of phenolic acids was 100 μM. Data are expressed as the means ± SEM of five independent determinations

Figure 5. Effect of phenolic acids of microbial origin on NAD-dependent respiration of mitochondria.

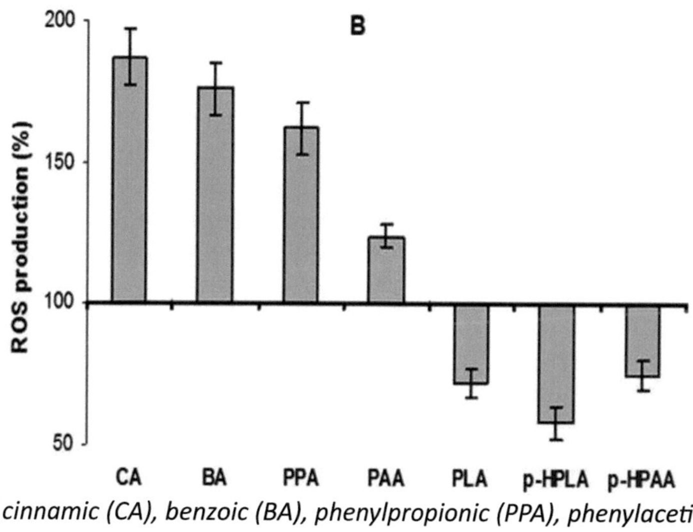

** cinnamic (CA), benzoic (BA), phenylpropionic (PPA), phenylacetic (PAA), p-hydroxyphenylpropionic (p-HPPA), phenyllactic (PLA), p-hydroxyphenyllactic (p-HPLA*

Data are expressed as means ± SEM of five independent determinations at a concentration of 100 μM

Figure 6. Comparison of the effect of phenolic acids* on menadione-activated ROS production by mitochondria.

When studying the effect of AMM on the production of ROS by mitochondria, activated by menadione, the differences were in the opposite direction: lipophilic AMM (cinnamic CA, benzoic BA, phenylpropionic PPA, and phenylacetic PAA) activated, and hydrophilic AMM (p-hydroxyphenyl propionic p-HPPA), phenyllactic PLA, and p-hydroxyphenyllactic p-HPLA opposite suppressed (**Figure 6**). It is known that a very large number of mitochondrial reactive oxygen species (mROS) directly damage proteins, lipids, and nucleic acids. At the same time, a complete lack of ROS production is also very harmful, so the lower levels of mROS are necessary for normal cell homeostasis. Low levels mROS perform the functions signaling molecules and need to adapt to the stress [35].

It is also shown the *in vitro* ability of microbial metabolites to influence the amount of metabolites of the tricarboxylic acid cycle in the blood of septic patients affects the activity of mitochondrial enzymes [36]. The clinical confirmation and significance of these facts to be assessed in the near future.

4.4. Hemodynamic instability and shock

Some authors view excessive bacterial load as the main cause of uncontrollable progression of hypotension in critically ill patients [37]. It has been shown that the earlier the onset of antimicrobial therapy (immediately on admission of a critical patient with signs of arterial hypotension) may have a significant impact on survival. So, hemodynamic instability and septic shock are undoubtedly connected with bacteria, but how? Attempts to explain the leading effect only of LPS (structural component of cell walls of gram-negative rods or endotoxin) is not satisfied, because they do not allow you to monitor and manage this process.

Our clinical monitoring of patients with high risk of septic shock indicates the potential involvement of AMM in the development of this life-threatening condition, accompanied by high mortality [38, 39]. In our view, an important role is played by disruption of the normal participation of microflora in the metabolism of aromatic amino acids, especially tyrosine and products of its metabolism. First, it is shown that an excess of toxic endogenous and microbial metabolic products of tyrosine and dopamine cannot be fully disposed of anaerobic microbiota [40]. However, these aromatic metabolites on the principle of feedback can inhibit the normal metabolic pathway of synthesis of hormones. Recently, we have obtained indirect evidence of "microbial" mechanism in the development of septic shock through the inhibition of tyrosine hydroxylase. In this way, the products of microbial metabolism may interfere with the normal synthesis of catecholamines from dopamine and to result in arterial hypotension. Search connection between endogenous hormones and bacterial exometabolites potentially related to hypotension in patients with infection will continue [41].

5. Conclusion

Sepsis integration of metabolism of humans and microbiota is disturbed and takes pathological character directed against the owner. Previously, it has been shown that phenyl carboxylic acids could have microbial origin in human blood of healthy people. Microbiota has to survive under adverse conditions, the indigenous anaerobic microflora are not able to fulfill its "helpful" metabolic functions [14]. Studies have shown that in septic patients, most violations occur in the metabolism of aromatic compounds. We documented imbalance of aromatic acids metabolites in septic patients: absence of serum PPA and high level of PLA, p-HPLA, and p-HPAA are associated with severity and mortality. Experimentally demonstrated the influence of some aromatic microbial metabolites (AMMs) on mitochondrial function, participate in the development of organ dysfunctions in sepsis. *In-vitro* some AMMs in clinically significant concentrations are able to inhibit phagocytic activity of neutrophils. Metabolism of tyrosine is severely disrupted in sepsis. Some microbial exometabolites may suppress the activity of enzymes such as tyrosine-hydroxylase. There is an excess of products of microbial biodegradation of endogenous metabolites of aromatic amino acids in the blood, including the reason of failure function of indigenous anaerobes. The obtained results indicate new promising target in the diagnosis, prevention, and treatment of sepsis.

We believe that the development of laboratory technologies, the use of other more sophisticated methods aimed at detection and measurement of metabolites of microbial origin in the human body, is the real path to success in solving the problem of sepsis in the near future.

6. Methods

We used gas chromatography-mass spectrometry (GC-MS) method to quantify metabolites in human serum from patients with pneumonia or abdomen sepsis, patients with local infection of the skin and soft tissues, healthy (as control). In the process, we adapted the sample preparation and measurement method for working in clinical laboratory conditions on GC-FID [42]. Clinical and laboratory data, APACHE II and SOFA scores in patients were matched. Methods for *in vitro* studies of the biological activity of microbial metabolites on the neutrophils and mitochondria are described in detail in articles listed in references. In microbiological experiments, we measured also the concentration of the metabolites by GH-MS in the nutrient medium after the cultivation of various species of aerobic or anaerobic bacteria. Data were compared by Mann-Whitney U-test; p-values less than 0.05 were considered significant.

Acknowledgements

I am grateful to my senior teachers, also to colleagues and associates in experimental and clinical work. This work was supported by the Russian Science Foundation Grant no. 15-15-00110.

Author details

Beloborodova Natalia Vladimirovna

Address all correspondence to: nvbeloborodova@yandex.ru

Federal Research and Clinical Center of Intensive Care Medicine and Rehabilitology, Negovsky Research Institute of General Reanimatology, Moscow, Russian Federation

References

[1] Tannock GW. Understanding the Gut Microbiota. John Wiley & Sons, Inc. Hoboken, New Jersey, - 184 p. ISBN 1118801342, 9781118801345

[2] Shenderov BA, Midtvedt T. Epigenomic programing: A future way to health? Microbial Ecology in Health & Disease 2014,**25**: 24145 - http://dx.doi.org/10.3402/mehd.v25.24145

[3] Beloborodova NV, Osipov GA. Homeostasis of small molecules originating from microbes and its role in microbial relations with the host. Vestnik Rossiiskoi Akademii Meditsinskikh Nauk. 1999;**54**(7):25-31. PMID: 10467881 https://www.ncbi.nlm.nih.gov/pubmed/10467881

[4] Wikoff WR, Anfora AT, Liu J, et al. Metabolomics analysis reveals large effects of gut microflora on mammalian blood metabolites. Proceedings of the National Academy of Sciences. 2009 March 10;**106**(10):3698-3703. DOI: 10.1073/pnas.0812874106

[5] Beloborodova NV, Osipov GA. Small molecules originating from microbes (SMOM) and their role in microbes–host relationship. Microbial Ecology in Health and Disease. 2000;**12**(1):12-21 http://www.microbecolhealthdis.net/index.php/mehd/article/view/8039

[6] Bianconi E, Piovesan A, Facchin F, Beraudi A, Casadei R, Frabetti F, et al. An estimation of the number of cells in the human body. Annals of Human Biology. 2013;**40**:463-471. DOI: 10.3109/03014460.2013.807878. pmid:23829164

[7] Sender R, Fuchs S, Milo R. Are we really vastly outnumbered? Revisiting the ratio of bacterial to host cells in humans. Cell. 2016;**164**:337-340. DOI: 10.1016/j.cell.2016.01.013. pmid:26824647

[8] Shimizu K, Ogura H, Goto M, Asahara T, Nomoto K, Morotomi M, Yoshiya K, Matsushima A, Sumi Y, Kuwagata Y, Tanaka H, Shimazu T, Sugimoto H. Altered gut flora and environment in patients with severe SIRS. Journal of Trauma. 2006;**60**(1):126-133. PMID: 16456446 DOI: 10.1097/01.ta.0000197374.99755.fe

[9] Kirsch M1. Bacterial overgrowth. American Journal of Gastroenterology. 1990 March; **85**(3):231-237. PMID: 2178395

[10] Beloborodova NV, Vostrikova TY, Antibiot Khimioter. Characteristics of fauces microflora in children treated in intensive care units. Article in Russian. 1998;**43**(8):16-22. PMID: 9777101

[11] Leeuwen PA, Boermeester MA, Houdijk AP, Ferwerda CC, Cuesta MA, Meyer S, Wesdorp RI. Clinical significance of translocation. Gut. 1994 January;**35**(Supp l):S28-S34. PMCID: PMC1378143

[12] Berg RD. Bacterial translocation from the gastrointestinal tract. Advances in Experimental Medicine and Biology. 1999;**473**:11-30. PMID: 10659341

[13] Deitch EA, Winterton J, Li M, Berg R. The gut as a portal of entry for bacteremia; role of protein malnutrition. Annals of Surgery. 1987 June;**205**(6):681-692

[14] Beloborodova NV. Integration of metabolism in man and his microbiome in critical conditions. General Reanimatology. 2012;**8**(4):42-54

[15] Beloborodova NV, Khodakova AS, Bairamov IT, Olenin AY. Microbial origin of phenylcarboxylic acids in the human body. Biochemistry (Moscow). 2009;**74**(12):1657-1663. PMID: 19961416 DOI: 10.1134/S0006297909120086 http://link.springer.com/article/10.1134/S0006297909120086

[16] Jenner AM, Rafter J, Halliwell B. Human faecal water content of phenolics: The extent of colonic exposure to aromatic compounds. Free Radical Biology & Medicine. 2005;**38**(6):763-772. DOI: 10.1016/j.freeradbiomed.2004.11.020

[17] Beloborodova NV, Moroz VV, Osipov AA, Bedova AY, Olenin AY, Getsina ML, Karpova OV, Olenina EG. Normal level of sepsis-associated phenylcarboxylic acids in human serum. Biochemistry (Moscow). 2015;**80**(3) 374-378. DOI: 10.1134/S0006297915030128, PMID: 25761691

[18] Beloborodova NV, Olenin AY, Khodakova AS, Chernevskaya EA, Khabib ON. Low-molecular phenol metabolites in blood serum: Origin and clinical significance. Anesteziologiya i Reanimatologiya. 2012;**5**:65-72

[19] Khodakova AS, Beloborodova NV. Microbial metabolites in the blood of patients with sepsis. Critical Care. 2007;**11**(4):P5. DOI: 10.1186/cc5984

[20] Beloborodova N, Osipov A, Pautova A, Bedova A. Aromatic metabolites clearance reflects the efficiency of ICU treatment more accurately then lactate clearance. Critical Care. 2016;**20**(Suppl 3):P19. DOI: 10.1186/s13054-016-1518-8

[21] Rogers AJ, McGeachie M, Baron RM, et al. Metabolomic derangements are associated with mortality in critically Ill adult patients. 2014; PLoS ONE **9**(1): e87538. DOI: 10.1371/journal.pone.0087538

[22] Sarshor YN, Beloborodova NV, Bedova AY, Osipov AA, Chernevskaya EA, Getsina ML. New criteria of bacterial load in critically ill patients. Shock. 2013;**40**(Suppl 1):31

[23] Beloborodova NV, Moroz VV, Bedova AY, Osipov AA, Sarshor YN,Chernevskaya EA. Participation of aromatic microbial metabolites in the development of severe infection and sepsis. Anesteziologiya i Reanimatologiya. 2016;**61**(3):202-208. DOI: 10.18821/0201-7563-2016-3-202-208

[24] Moroz VV, Beloborodova NV, Osipov AA, Vlasenko AV, Bedova AY, Pautova AK. Phenylcarboxylic acids in the assessment of the severity of patient condition and the efficiency of intensive treatment in critical care medicine. Obshchaya Reanimatologiya. 2016;**12**(4):37-48. http://www.reanimatology.com/rmt/article/view/1538 DOI: 10.15360/1813-9779-2016-4-37-48.

[25] Beloborodova N, Bairamov I, Olenin A, Shubina V, Teplova V, Fedotcheva N. Effect of phenolic acids of microbial origin on production of reactive oxygen species in mitochondria and neutrophils. Journal of Biomedical Science. 2012;**19**:89. DOI: 10.1186/1423-0127-19-89

[26] Vincent JL, Nelson DR, Williams MD. Is worsening multiple organ failure the cause of death in patients with severe sepsis? Critical Care Medicine. 2011;**39**(5):1050-1055. DOI: 10.1097/CCM.0b013e31820eda29

[27] Hotchkiss RS, Karl IE. The pathophysiology and treatment of sepsis. The New England Journal of Medicine. 2003 January 9;**348**(2):138-150. DOI: 10.1056/NEJMra021333

[28] Abraham E, Singer M. Mechanisms of sepsis-induced organ dysfunction. Critical Care Medicine. 2007 October;**35**(10):2408-2416

[29] Singer M. Cellular dysfunction in sepsis. Clinics in Chest Medicine. 2008 December; **29**(4):655-660. PMID:18954700. DOI: 10.1016/j.ccm.2008.06.003

[30] Friedman JR, Nunnari J. Mitochondrial form and function. Nature. 2014;**505**:335-343

[31] Exline MC, Crouser ED. Mitochondrial mechanisms of sepsis-induced organ failure. Frontiers in Bioscience. 2008 May 1;**13**:5030-5041. Review. PMID: 18508567 https://www.ncbi.nlm.nih.gov/pmc/articles/PMC3913468

[32] Singer M. The role of mitochondrial dysfunction in sepsis-induced multi-organ failure Virulence. 2014 January 1;**5**(1):66-72. PMCID: PMC3916385 DOI: 10.4161/viru.26907

[33] Beloborodova NV, Teplova VV, Fedotcheva NI. Monograph: The Role of Microbial Metabolites in Mitochondrial Dysfunction in Sepsis. Germany: LAP Lambert Academic Publishing; 2013. p. 89. ISBN: 978-3-659-43111-1 (translation)

[34] Fedotcheva NI, Kazakov RE, Kondrashova MN, Beloborodova NV. Toxic effects of microbial phenolic acids on the functions of mitochondria. Toxicology Letters. 2008 August 28;**180**(3):182-188. DOI: 10.1016/j.toxlet.2008.06.861

[35] Sena LA, Chandel NS. Physiological roles of mitochondrial reactive oxygen species molecular. Cell. 2012 October 26;**48(**2):158-167. DOI: http://dx.doi.org/10.1016/j.molcel.2012.09.025

[36] Fedotcheva NI, Litvinova EG, Osipov AA, Olenin AY, Moroz VV, Beloborodova NV. Influence of microbial metabolites of phenolic nature on the activity of mitochondrial enzymes. Biophysics. 2015;6:IF-0.316. PMID:26841505

[37] Kumar A, Roberts D, Wood KE, Light B, Parrillo JE, Sharma S, Suppes R, Feinstein D, Zanotti S, Taiberg L, Gurka D, Kumar A, Cheang M. Duration of hypotension before initiation of effective antimicrobial therapy is the critical determinant of survival in human septic shock. Critical Care Medicine. 2006;**34**:1589-1596. DOI: 10.1097/01.CCM.0000217961.75225.E9

[38] Beloborodova NV, Sarshor YN, Bedova AY, Pautova AK, Chernevskaya EA. Are phenyllactic and p-hydroxyphenyllactic acids involved in the development of arterial hypotension? Infection. 2015;**43**(Suppl 1):S31. DOI: 10.1007/s15010-015-0827-1

[39] Sarshor Y, Beloborodova N, Moroz V, Osipov A, Bedova A, Chernevskaya E, Getsina M. Value of microbial metabolites in blood serum as criteria for bacterial load in the pathogenesis of hemodynamic disorders in critically ill patients. Critical Care. 2014;18(Suppl 1):P208. DOI:10.1186/cc13398 http://ccforum.com/content/18/S1/P208

[40] Beloborodova N, Moroz V, Osipov A, Bedova A, Sarshor Y, Vlasenko A, Olenin A. Tyrosine metabolism disorder and the potential capability of anaerobic microbiota to decrease the value of aromatic metabolites in critically ill patients. Critical Care. 2014;18(Suppl 2):P60. DOI: 10.1186/cc14063 http://ccforum.com/content/18/S2/P60

[41] Beloborodova NV, Chernevskaya EA, Bedova AY, Sarshor YN, Sergeev AA. Connection between aromatic microbial metabolites, hormones and biomarkers in critically ill patients with infection. Shock. 2016;**46**(Suppl 2):P1-9

[42] Moroz V, Beloborodova NV, Bedova AY, Revel'skii AI, Getsina ML, Osipov AA, Sarshor YN, Buchinskaya AA, Olenin AY. Development of methods of the gas chromatographic determination of phenylcarboxylic acids in blood serum and their adaptation to clinical laboratory conditions. Journal of Analytical Chemistry. 2015 April;**70**(4):495-501. DOI: 10.1134/S1061934815040103

Section 2

Age and Sepsis

Chapter 2

Septic Shock in Older People

Mike Yoshio Hamasaki,

Marcel Cerqueira César Machado and

Fabiano Pinheiro da Silva

Additional information is available at the end of the chapter

http://dx.doi.org/10.5772/68080

Abstract

Sepsis is a complex condition that is initiated by infection. The incidence of sepsis and its severity are higher at an older age (mean age of approximately 65 years). Clinical manifestations of sepsis are derived from systemic inflammatory response syndrome. Age-related defects in immunity are shown by changes in cellular and humoral immunity. Recent studies have shown significant changes in the innate response (e.g., changes in toll-like receptor expression, abnormal activation of mitogen-activated protein kinases, and production of reactive oxygen species) in older people. Transcriptomic analysis on a large scale has provided interesting information showing that specific groups of patients actually have singular profiles for inflammatory responses. Findings from our research group have identified major molecular pathways that are particularly affected in older people during sepsis. Oxidative phosphorylation pathways and mitochondrial dysfunction are altered the most in older people with sepsis compared with younger patients with sepsis. These pathways might have a pivotal role in worsening clinical outcomes compared with younger people with sepsis. The mechanisms leading to specific dysfunction of several signaling pathways in the immune response of older people are complex and appear to involve multiple factors, including environmental factors, microRNAs, and epigenetic changes.

Keywords: sepsis, aging, inflammation, transcriptomics

1. Introduction

Sepsis is a complex disease that is triggered by infection and characterized by massive deregulation of the immune system [1]. Clinical manifestations of sepsis, such as fever, a hypercoagulable

INTECH
open science | open minds

© 2017 The Author(s). Licensee InTech. This chapter is distributed under the terms of the Creative Commons Attribution License (http://creativecommons.org/licenses/by/3.0), which permits unrestricted use, distribution, and reproduction in any medium, provided the original work is properly cited.

state, and peripheral hypotension, are derived from systemic inflammatory response syndrome (SIRS). Clinically, SIRS can be classified according to the nature of the symptoms manifested by the individual, such as (1) hypothermia or fever, (2) tachycardia, (3) tachypnea, and (4) leukocytosis or leucopenia [2]. Infection is probably the most common cause of SIRS, associated with the action of cytokines that are derived from cells of the immune system acting in organs and systems with specific receptors [3]. **Figure 1** illustrates the stages of evolution of sepsis using SIRS as the standard diagnosis.

Recently, the Journal of the American Medical Association (JAMA) published the "Third International Consensus Definitions for Sepsis and Septic Shock (Sepsis-3)." This is the most recent international consensus on diagnostic criteria for sepsis and septic shock. According to the new criteria for the diagnosis of sepsis, organ dysfunction promoted by the disease must be considered [4]. In this regard, SIRS is no longer used as a diagnostic criterion for sepsis, and organ dysfunction is represented by an increase of two or more points in the Sequential Organ Failure Assessment (SOFA) score. The SOFA score is obtained by using a scoring scheme that assigns one to four points. The SOFA score uses variables, such as the platelet count, bilirubin, and oxygenation index, using variables as scoring of platelet, bilirubin, oxygenation index, use of vasoactive drugs, the Glasgow Coma Scale, and creatinine.

Septic patients have an average age of approximately 65 years [5], and the incidence of sepsis and its severity are significantly increased at an older age [6, 7]. Factors that contribute to this increase include defects in the integrity of epithelial barriers, dysfunction in the cough reflex, changes in level of consciousness, immobility, comorbidities, presence of invasive medical devices, a decrease in physiological reserves, endocrine disorders, and malnutrition [8, 9].

Immune defects associated with age are shown by changes in cellular and humoral immunity [10]. Aging is associated with an increase in memory T-cell [9] repertoire and in the responses of types 1 and 2 [11, 12]. B cells gradually decrease with age, while the production of immunoglobulin increases [13].

Initial reports described preservation of the innate immune response in older people [14], but recent studies have shown significant changes in these components [9]. Studies have

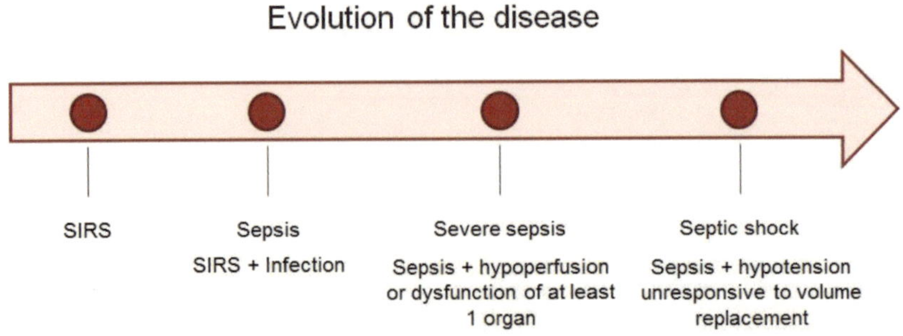

Figure 1. Evolution of sepsis.

suggested changes in expression and toll-like receptor (TLR) function as age advances and that this affects the response to pathogens [15]. An increase in the basal levels of inflammatory mediators [16, 17], aberrant activation of mitogen-activated protein kinases [18], an increased number of apoptotic cells [19], defects in the process of phagocytosis, production of reactive oxygen species (ROS), and deregulation in expression of accessory molecules have been reported [20]. Indeed, evidence indicates that older people produce higher levels of pro-inflammatory cytokines, coagulation factors, and acute phase proteins in the absence of infection [21–23].

However, the inflammatory response of older people in the presence of a serious infectious process remains controversial. Because of the increasing aging population, this issue has received great attention from the scientific community (**Figure 2**). Studies have identified a higher mortality, inflammatory response, hypothermia, disseminated intravascular coagulation, and apoptosis in aged animals undergoing experimental models of sepsis [24]. Aspects

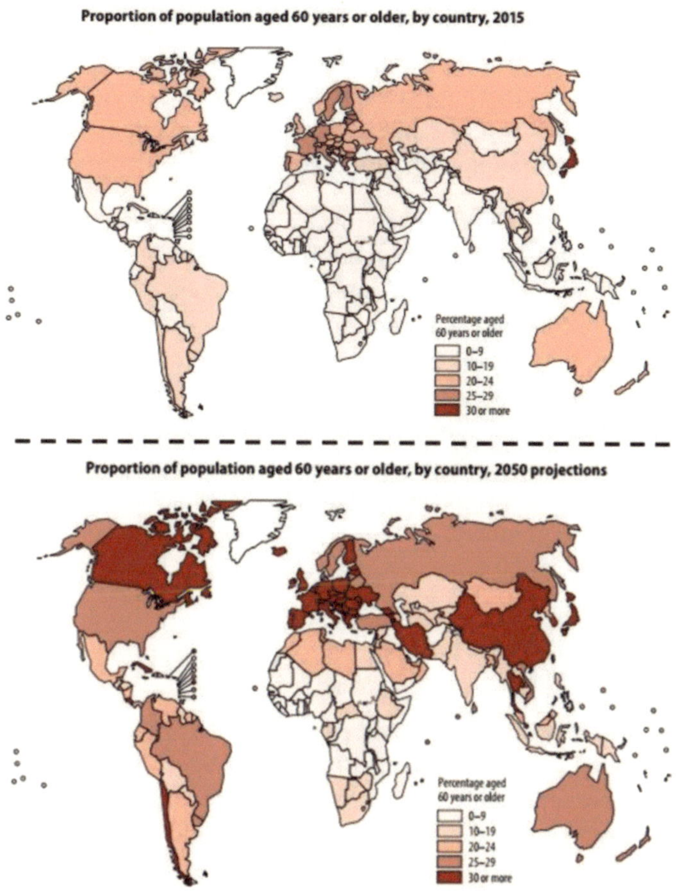

Figure 2. Population aging around the world. Source: World Health Organization—World report on Ageing and Health —2015.

of immunosenescence and a more intense inflammatory response in aged rodents with sepsis have been well characterized [25, 26]. However, intriguingly, clinical studies (including our own research group) have detected a similar immune response profile when comparing older patients with sepsis with younger patients [27–30].

2. Transcriptomics in sepsis

Transcriptomics is a powerful technique, which can be used for detecting new therapeutic biomarkers and targets in the field of infectious diseases [31, 32]. Several studies of gene expression in sepsis on a large scale have been performed. These studies have shown persistent repression of genes of adaptive immunity and massive activation of pathways of innate immunity in septic shock [33]. Using RNA obtained from total blood, Wong and colleagues [34] identified activation of oxidative phosphorylation, signaling by interleukin (IL)-10, TLRs, TREM, NF-κB, the protein ubiquitination pathway, and IL-6 in macrophages. These authors also described suppression of specific pathways of T lymphocytes and signaling by chemokines (CCR5). Similarly, Cvijanovich and colleagues [35] detected activation of TLRs, IL-10, IL-6, and NF-κB with concomitant suppression of T lymphocytes. Additionally, they detected activation of protein in the acute phase, p38, the complement system, and some nuclear receptors (LXR and PPAR) in association with repression of antigenic presentation pathways.

Shanley et al. [36] used total blood RNA from septic patients and performed global gene expression experiments. Their results agree with those studies described above in many aspects, except that they also identified integrin activation, IGF-1, GM-CSF, and insulin receiver. Tang et al. [37] described activation of apoptosis genes, including *CARD12*, *APAF1*, and *ELMOD2*, in mononuclear cells of septic patients. Moreover, a recent study in patients with severe blunt trauma described surprisingly similar results with activation of a large number of genes involved in inflammation, pattern recognition, and antimicrobial function [38]. This study also showed simultaneous repression of genes involved in antigenic presentation and proliferation of T cells, suggesting that severe physiological stress, regardless of the cause, has similar genetic signatures.

3. Sepsis: a heterogeneous disease

Sepsis affects different groups of patients (e.g., those with an older age, diabetes, nephropathy, multiple trauma, surgery, and obesity). Historically, each specific group of patients is thought to be present with a characteristic inflammatory response. In the course of sepsis, transition of the inflammatory response to standard immunosuppression has been suggested to explain the disappointing results obtained by clinical studies that investigated the use of anti-inflammatory drugs in this population of patients [39–41]. Transcriptomic analysis on a large scale has provided interesting information in this regard, showing that specific groups of patients actually have singular profiles [42–44]. However, a recently published systematic review was unable to detect distinct pro-inflammatory and anti-inflammatory phases in sepsis or differences in gene expression when analyzing different sub-populations [45]. Therefore, this issue remains extremely controversial.

To the best of our knowledge, our research group was the first to study characteristics of sepsis in older people through transcriptomics analysis on a large scale [46]. We detected 388 genes that were differentially expressed between older and younger people with sepsis and 442 genes among older and healthy younger subjects.

Interestingly, oxidative phosphorylation pathways and mitochondrial dysfunction were the most altered in older people with sepsis compared with younger patients with sepsis. Other relevant pathways were signaling by TGF-β, Wnt/β-catenin, and calcium, as well as pathways that have been less studied in this disease, such as those involved in nerve growth factor and bone morphogenic protein.

Initially, our results confirmed that, regarding the production of TNF-α, IL-6, IL-1β, TLRs, and other classical markers of cell activation, younger and older people respond similarly to a severe infectious insult. Some other pathways, as described above, appear to be more affected in older patients in a critical condition than in younger patients. We consider that defects of mitochondrial function and oxidative phosphorylation, and signaling by TGF-β, Wnt/β-catenin, bone morphogenic protein, nerve growth factor, and calcium are different in older patients with sepsis than in younger patients with sepsis.

Confirming our hypothesis, we observed a notable decrease in gene expression of the mitochondrial respiratory chain in older patients with sepsis [46]. Mitochondrial dysfunction is known for contributing to multiple organ failure in sepsis. Physiologically, small amounts of reactive species of oxygen are produced by complex I and III of the respiratory chain. Sepsis is characterized by an increase in oxidative stress due to increased production of neutrophils, an increase in xanthine oxidase activity, increased plasma levels of nitric oxide, and decreased antioxidant capacity of plasma [47]. Pro-inflammatory mediators and oxidative stress deregulate the function of respiratory chain enzymes and lead to structural damage of lipids, proteins, and mitochondrial DNA [48, 49], promoting failure of multiple organs [50]. Mitochondrial damage and secondary dysfunction to oxidative stress are also characteristic of the aging process [6, 51, 52]. Mice that have defective function of mitochondrial DNA polymerase enzyme have a shorter life and show many signs of premature aging, such as alopecia, decreased physical activity, and early loss of reproductive function [53].

The mechanisms that lead to specific dysfunction of several signaling pathways in the immune response of older people are complex and involve multiple factors. We propose that environmental factors [54, 55], microRNAs [56], and epigenetic changes [57] play a major role in modulating the immune response cascades that are particularly affected in older patients.

Our data confirm previous reports that aging is accompanied by changes in gene expression of immune system pathways [58]. Another important result of our research group shows that noncoding long RNA subgroups are deregulated in sepsis and during the aging process.

Therefore, extensive studies are required to investigate the biological role played by this class of transcripts in septic shock in older individuals.

4. Conclusion

There is great expectation that studying biological systems can provide a better understanding of several complex diseases. Further information could be used to identify new therapeutic targets and groups of patients who should benefit from such interventions.

Using this strategy, we have identified the main pathways that are altered in older people with sepsis. Our findings highlight that the systemic inflammatory response differs depending on the population that is studied. Oxidative stress appears to play a central role, inducing various types of dysfunction, in older patients with sepsis. Moreover, we have identified several other genes and signaling pathways that are altered in these patients. This information will facilitate understanding of the nature of the immune response in this situation.

Author details

Mike Yoshio Hamasaki, Marcel Cerqueira César Machado and Fabiano Pinheiro da Silva*

*Address all correspondence to: pinheirofabiano@hotmail.com

Emergency Medicine Department, University of São Paulo, Brazil

References

[1] Iskander KN, Osuchowski MF, Stearns-Kurosawa DJ, Kurosawa S, Stepien D, Valentine C, et al. Sepsis: multiple abnormalities, heterogeneous responses, and evolving understanding. Physiol Rev. 2013;93(3):1247-88.

[2] Levy MM, Fink MP, Marshall JC, Abraham E, Angus D, Cook D, et al. 2001 SCCM/ESICM/ACCP/ATS/SIS International Sepsis Definitions Conference. Crit Care Med. 2003;31(4):1250-6.

[3] Yao YM, Luan YY, Zhang QH, Sheng ZY. Pathophysiological aspects of sepsis: an overview. Methods Mol Biol. 2015;1237:5-15.

[4] Singer M, Deutschman CS, Seymour CW, Shankar-Hari M, Annane D, Bauer M, et al. The Third International Consensus Definitions for Sepsis and Septic Shock (Sepsis-3). JAMA. 2016;315(8):801-10.

[5] De Gaudio AR, Rinaldi S, Chelazzi C, Borracci T. Pathophysiology of sepsis in the elderly: clinical impact and therapeutic considerations. Curr Drug Targets. 2009;10(1):60-70.

[6] Opal SM, Girard TD, Ely EW. The immunopathogenesis of sepsis in elderly patients. Clin Infect Dis. 2005;41(Suppl 7):S504-12.

[7] Heppner HJ, Cornel S, Peter W, Philipp B, Katrin S. Infections in the elderly. Crit Care Clin. 2013;29(3):757-74.

[8] Nasa P, Juneja D, Singh O. Severe sepsis and septic shock in the elderly: An overview. World J Crit Care Med. 2012;1(1):23-30.

[9] Girard TD, Opal SM, Ely EW. Insights into severe sepsis in older patients: from epidemiology to evidence-based management. Clin Infect Dis. 2005;40(5):719-27.

[10] Grubeck-Loebenstein B, Wick G. The aging of the immune system. Adv Immunol. 2002;80:243-84.

[11] Plackett TP, Schilling EM, Faunce DE, Choudhry MA, Witte PL, Kovacs EJ. Aging enhances lymphocyte cytokine defects after injury. FASEB J. 2003;17(6):688-9.

[12] Mascarucci P, Taub D, Saccani S, Paloma MA, Dawson H, Roth GS, et al. Age-related changes in cytokine production by leukocytes in rhesus monkeys. Aging (Milano). 2001;13(2):85-94.

[13] Weksler ME, Goodhardt M, Szabo P. The effect of age on B cell development and humoral immunity. Springer Semin Immunopathol. 2002;24(1):35-52.

[14] Shinkai S, Konishi M, Shephard RJ. Aging and immune response to exercise. Can J Physiol Pharmacol. 1998;76(5):562-72.

[15] Renshaw M, Rockwell J, Engleman C, Gewirtz A, Katz J, Sambhara S. Cutting edge: impaired Toll-like receptor expression and function in aging. J Immunol. 2002;169(9): 4697-701.

[16] Shaw AC, Goldstein DR, Montgomery RR. Age-dependent dysregulation of innate immunity. Nat Rev Immunol. 2013;13(12):875-87.

[17] Howcroft TK, Campisi J, Louis GB, Smith MT, Wise B, Wyss-Coray T, et al. The role of inflammation in age-related disease. Aging (Albany NY). 2013;5(1):84-93.

[18] Boehmer ED, Goral J, Faunce DE, Kovacs EJ. Age-dependent decrease in Toll-like receptor 4-mediated proinflammatory cytokine production and mitogen-activated protein kinase expression. J Leukoc Biol. 2004;75(2):342-9.

[19] Plackett TP, Boehmer ED, Faunce DE, Kovacs EJ. Aging and innate immune cells. J Leukoc Biol. 2004;76(2):291-9.

[20] Franceschi C, Bonafe M, Valensin S. Human immunosenescence: the prevailing of innate immunity, the failing of clonotypic immunity, and the filling of immunological space. Vaccine. 2000;18(16):1717-20.

[21] Fagiolo U, Cossarizza A, Scala E, Fanales-Belasio E, Ortolani C, Cozzi E, et al. Increased cytokine production in mononuclear cells of healthy elderly people. Eur J Immunol. 1993;23(9):2375-8.

[22] Mari D, Mannucci PM, Coppola R, Bottasso B, Bauer KA, Rosenberg RD. Hypercoagulability in centenarians: the paradox of successful aging. Blood. 1995;85(11): 3144-9.

[23] Cevenini E, Monti D, Franceschi C. Inflammageing. Curr Opin Clin Nutr Metab Care. 2013;16(1):14-20.

[24] Starr ME, Saito H. Sepsis in old age: review of human and animal studies. Aging Dis. 2014;5(2):126-36.

[25] Tateda K, Matsumoto T, Miyazaki S, Yamaguchi K. Lipopolysaccharide-induced lethality and cytokine production in aged mice. Infect Immun. 1996;64(3):769-74.

[26] Turnbull IR, Wlzorek JJ, Osborne D, Hotchkiss RS, Coopersmith CM, Buchman TG. Effects of age on mortality and antibiotic efficacy in cecal ligation and puncture. Shock. 2003;19(4):310-3.

[27] Pinheiro da Silva F, Zampieri FG, Barbeiro DF, Barbeiro HV, Goulart AC, Torggler Filho F, et al. Septic shock in older people: a prospective cohort study. Immun Ageing. 2013;10(1):21.

[28] Kale S, Yende S, Kong L, Perkins A, Kellum JA, Newman AB, et al. The effects of age on inflammatory and coagulation-fibrinolysis response in patients hospitalized for pneumonia. PLoS One. 2010;5(11):e13852.

[29] Kelly E, MacRedmond RE, Cullen G, Greene CM, McElvaney NG, O'Neill SJ. Community-acquired pneumonia in older patients: does age influence systemic cytokine levels in community-acquired pneumonia? Respirology. 2009;14(2):210-6.

[30] Kale SS, Yende S. Effects of Aging on Inflammation and Hemostasis through the Continuum of Critical Illness. Aging Dis. 2011;2(6):501-11.

[31] Chaussabel D, Pascual V, Banchereau J. Assessing the human immune system through blood transcriptomics. BMC Biol. 2010;8:84.

[32] Christie JD. Microarrays. Crit Care Med. 2005;33(12 Suppl):S449-52.

[33] Wong HR, Cvijanovich N, Allen GL, Lin R, Anas N, Meyer K, et al. Genomic expression profiling across the pediatric systemic inflammatory response syndrome, sepsis, and septic shock spectrum. Crit Care Med. 2009;37(5):1558-66.

[34] Wong HR, Freishtat RJ, Monaco M, Odoms K, Shanley TP. Leukocyte subset-derived genomewide expression profiles in pediatric septic shock. Pediatr Crit Care Med. 2010;11(3):349-55.

[35] Cvijanovich N, Shanley TP, Lin R, Allen GL, Thomas NJ, Checchia P, et al. Validating the genomic signature of pediatric septic shock. Physiol Genomics. 2008;34(1):127-34.

[36] Shanley TP, Cvijanovich N, Lin R, Allen GL, Thomas NJ, Doctor A, et al. Genome-level longitudinal expression of signaling pathways and gene networks in pediatric septic shock. Mol Med. 2007;13(9-10):495-508.

[37] Tang BM, McLean AS, Dawes IW, Huang SJ, Lin RC. Gene-expression profiling of peripheral blood mononuclear cells in sepsis. Crit Care Med. 2009;37(3):882-8.

[38] Xiao W, Mindrinos MN, Seok J, Cuschieri J, Cuenca AG, Gao H, et al. A genomic storm in critically injured humans. J Exp Med. 2011;208(13):2581-90.

[39] Bone RC. Sir Isaac Newton, sepsis, SIRS, and CARS. Crit Care Med. 1996;24(7):1125-8.

[40] Bone RC. Why sepsis trials fail. JAMA. 1996;276(7):565-6.

[41] Bone RC, Grodzin CJ, Balk RA. Sepsis: a new hypothesis for pathogenesis of the disease process. Chest. 1997;112(1):235-43.

[42] Maslove DM, Wong HR. Gene expression profiling in sepsis: timing, tissue, and translational considerations. Trends Mol Med. 2014;20(4):204-13.

[43] Maslove DM, Tang BM, McLean AS. Identification of sepsis subtypes in critically ill adults using gene expression profiling. Crit Care. 2012;16(5):R183.

[44] Severino P, Silva E, Baggio-Zappia GL, Brunialti MK, Nucci LA, Rigato O, Jr., et al. Patterns of gene expression in peripheral blood mononuclear cells and outcomes from patients with sepsis secondary to community acquired pneumonia. PLoS One. 2014;9(3):e91886.

[45] Tang BM, Huang SJ, McLean AS. Genome-wide transcription profiling of human sepsis: a systematic review. Crit Care. 2010;14(6):R237.

[46] Pellegrina DVS, Severino P, Barbeiro HV, Andreghetto FM, Velasco IT, Souza HP, et al. Septic shock in advanced age: transcriptome analysis reveals altered molecular signatures in neutrophil granulocytes. PLoS One 2015;10(6):e0128341.

[47] Wendel M, Heller AR. Mitochondrial function and dysfunction in sepsis. Wien Med Wochenschr. 2010;160(5-6):118-23.

[48] Suliman HB, Carraway MS, Piantadosi CA. Postlipopolysaccharide oxidative damage of mitochondrial DNA. Am J Respir Crit Care Med. 2003;167(4):570-9.

[49] Garcia-Ruiz C, Colell A, Mari M, Morales A, Fernandez-Checa JC. Direct effect of ceramide on the mitochondrial electron transport chain leads to generation of reactive oxygen species. Role of mitochondrial glutathione. J Biol Chem. 1997;272(17):11369-77.

[50] Galley HF. Oxidative stress and mitochondrial dysfunction in sepsis. Br J Anaesth. 2011;107(1):57-64.

[51] Cannizzo ES, Clement CC, Sahu R, Follo C, Santambrogio L. Oxidative stress, inflam-maging and immunosenescence. J Proteomics. 2011;74(11):2313-23.

[52] Floyd RA, Towner RA, He T, Hensley K, Maples KR. Translational research involving oxidative stress and diseases of aging. Free Radic Biol Med. 2011;51(5):931-41.

[53] Trifunovic A, Wredenberg A, Falkenberg M, Spelbrink JN, Rovio AT, Bruder CE, et al. Premature ageing in mice expressing defective mitochondrial DNA polymerase. Nature. 2004;429(6990):417-23.

[54] Su DM, Aw D, Palmer DB. Immunosenescence: a product of the environment? Curr Opin Immunol. 2013;25(4):498-503.

[55] Muller L, Pawelec G. Aging and immunity impact of behavioral intervention. Brain Behav Immun. 2014;39:8-22.

[56] Harries LW. MicroRNAs as mediators of the ageing process. Genes (Basel). 2014;5(3): 656-70.

[57] Weidner CI, Wagner W. The epigenetic tracks of aging. Biol Chem. 2014.

[58] de Magalhaes JP, Curado J, Church GM. Meta-analysis of age-related gene expression profiles identifies common signatures of aging. Bioinformatics. 2009;25(7):875-81.

Section 3

Host Inhibitory Mechansim in Sepsis

Chapter 3

Kallistatin in Sepsis: Protective Actions and Potential Therapeutic Applications

Julie Chao, Pengfei Li and Lee Chao

Additional information is available at the end of the chapter

http://dx.doi.org/10.5772/67988

Abstract

Sepsis is a systemic inflammatory response to infection, leading to multiorgan injury and mortality. Kallistatin is an endogenous protein expressed in the liver and tissues relevant to cardiovascular function. Kallistatin levels are markedly reduced in patients with sepsis and liver disease and in lipopolysaccharide (LPS)-induced septic mice. Kallistatin administration attenuates inflammation, multiorgan damage, and lethality in septic mice with LPS treatment, group A streptococcal, or polymicrobial infection. Importantly, kallistatin treatment not only prevents but also reverses organ injury and lethality in septic mice. Kallistatin decreases sepsis-induced inflammatory responses and tissue damage by modulating differential signaling pathways, including: (1) stimulating endothelial nitric oxide (eNOS) and sirtuin 1 (SIRT) synthesis, and NO formation; (2) increasing suppressor of cytokine signaling-3 (SOCS3) expression; (3) antagonizing tumor necrosis factor-α (TNF-α) and high mobility group box 1 (HMGB1)-mediated oxidative stress and inflammatory gene expression; and (4) displaying bactericidal effects by stimulating superoxide formation. Therefore, kallistatin's multifactorial activities provide effective protection during septic shock in animal models. As kallistatin displays no apparent cytotoxicity, kallistatin therapy may provide a promising approach for the treatment of sepsis in humans.

Keywords: kallistatin, sepsis, oxidative stress, inflammation, organ injury

1. Introduction

Sepsis is a major contributor to the morbidity and mortality of intensive care patients and a leading cause of death worldwide [1, 2]. Sepsis is a systemic inflammatory response to infection that can lead to multiorgan dysfunction and is mediated by both early (tumor necrosis factor-α, TNF-α) and late (high mobility group box 1, HMGB1) inflammatory cytokines [2, 3]. Although the underlying pathophysiology of sepsis has not been completely elucidated,

INTECH
open science | open minds

© 2017 The Author(s). Licensee InTech. This chapter is distributed under the terms of the Creative Commons Attribution License (http://creativecommons.org/licenses/by/3.0), which permits unrestricted use, distribution, and reproduction in any medium, provided the original work is properly cited.

TNF-α and HMGB1 upregulation is known to play a critical role in the inflammatory response [4–6]. Moreover, suppressor of cytokine signaling-3 (SOCS3), a feedback inhibitor of lipopolysaccharide (LPS)-induced inflammation, has been shown to be a key player in inhibiting nuclear factor (NF)-κB–mediated pro-inflammatory cytokine production [7–9]. Anti-inflammatory strategies have been investigated with favorable effects in animal models of sepsis but with marginal results in humans [10]. Consequently, clinical trials for sepsis have been referred to as the "graveyard for pharmaceutical companies" [10]. Because numerous signaling cascades are triggered during septic shock, selective blocking of inflammatory mediators is not sufficient to arrest this process. Therefore, the development of novel strategies is vital to the effective treatment of sepsis patients.

Kallistatin was first identified in human plasma as a tissue kallikrein-binding protein (KBP) and a new serine proteinase inhibitor (serpin) [11–13]. Kallistatin modulates a wide spectrum of biological activities independent of tissue kallikrein [14–20]. Kallistatin is mainly expressed in the liver but is also present in the heart, kidney, and blood vessel [21–23]. Kallistatin protein contains two structural elements: an active site and a heparin-binding domain [24–26]. The active site of kallistatin is necessary for complex formation with tissue kallikrein and thus inhibition of tissue kallikrein activity and bioavailability [13, 27]. Kallistatin's heparin-binding domain, however, is essential for antagonizing signaling pathways mediated by vascular endothelial growth factor (VEGF), TNF-α, HMGB1, and transforming growth factor (TGF)-β [16, 20, 28, 29]. Kallistatin levels are markedly reduced in hypertensive or normotensive rodents with cardiac and renal injury or streptozotocin-induced diabetes [11, 18, 30–32]. Circulatory kallistatin levels are also diminished in patients with liver disease, septic syndrome, diabetic retinopathy, severe pneumonia, inflammatory bowel disease, obesity, prostate, and colon cancer [33–40]. Kallistatin administration by gene or protein delivery protects against the pathogenesis of hypertension, heart and kidney damage, arthritis, influenza virus infection, tumor growth, and metastasis in animal models [15–19, 41–46]. Conversely, depletion of endogenous kallistatin by neutralizing antibody injection exacerbates cardiovascular and renal injury in hypertensive rats [47]. These findings indicate that kallistatin modulates a wide spectrum of biological activities, such as blood pressure, inflammation, multiorgan injury, and cancer.

2. Kallistatin via its structural elements regulates differential signaling pathways

Kallistatin through its two functional domains modulates numerous signaling pathways and biological activities. Kallistatin's active site is crucial for: (1) complex formation with tissue kallikrein and inhibiting tissue kallikrein activity and bioavailability [13, 27]; (2) increasing eNOS and SIRT1 expression and activation, leading to elevated NO formation [28]; (3) stimulating SOCS3 expression [48]; and (4) interacting with a tyrosine kinase [28, 48]. Kallistatin via its heparin-binding domain interacts with cell surface heparan sulfate proteoglycans, thereby antagonizing the following biological effects: (1) VEGF-mediated angiogenesis and vascular permeability [16, 20]; (2) TNF-α–induced NF-κB activation, inflammation, oxidative stress, and apoptosis [20]; (3) HMGB1-induced inflammatory gene expression and oxidative stress [29]; (4) TGF-β–induced endothelial-mesenchymal transition (EndMT), and epithelial-mesenchymal transition (EMT) [28]; (5) Wnt-mediated cancer cell proliferation, migration, invasion, and autophagy [42, 44]; and (6) EGF-induced cancer cell migration and invasion (unpublished results). Thus, kallistatin, with its multifactorial activities, regulates a wide spectrum of biological processes, such as angiogenesis, inflammation, oxidative stress, apoptosis, fibrosis, and cancer development.

3. Depleted kallistatin expression and levels in organ damage and sepsis

Kallistatin is a member of the serpin family, which also includes α1-antitrypsin and α1-antichymotrypsisn [21]. In contrast to α1-antitrypsin, kallistatin is a negative acute-phase protein, as kallistatin expression in rat liver is rapidly downregulated within 24 h after lipopolysaccharide (LPS)-induced endotoxemia [31]. Kallistatin levels are depleted in animal models with hypertension, diabetes, cardiovascular, and renal damage [11, 18, 29–31]. Circulatory kallistatin levels are markedly reduced in patients with septic syndrome, liver disease, diabetic retinopathy, inflammatory bowel disease, and severe pneumonia [33, 34, 36–38]. LPS (endotoxin) from Gram-negative bacteria, or peptidoglycan (PepG) and lipoteichoic acid (LTA) from Gram-positive bacteria, are capable of inducing TNF-α synthesis and reactive oxygen species (ROS) formation [49–54]. TNF-α stimulates ROS information in endothelial cells and endothelial progenitor cells [17, 43, 55, 56]. Kallistatin expression and levels are negatively regulated by H_2O_2 through JNK-dependent FOXO1 activation in endothelial cells [57]. Like ROS, TNF-α dramatically suppresses kallistatin expression in endothelial cells (**Figure 1A**). Therefore, kallistatin levels are depleted by the activation of the TNF-α–ROS signaling pathway during septic shock (**Figure 1B**).

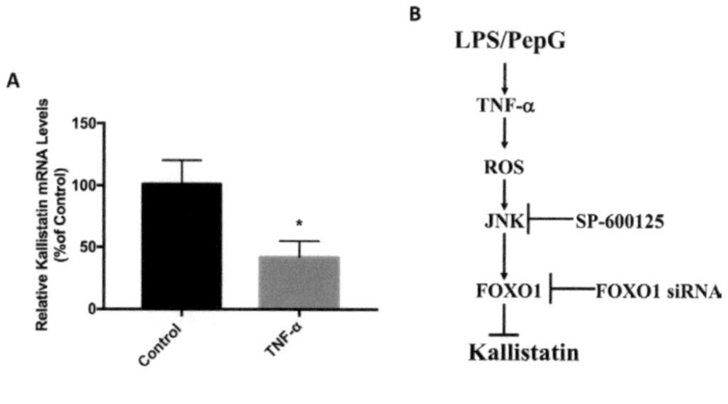

Figure 1. (A) TNF-α inhibits kallistatin expression in endothelial cells. TNF-α (10 ng/ml) significantly decreases kallistatin expression in endothelial cells. $n = 3$, *$P < 0.05$ vs. control groups. (B) LPS/PepG exposure leads to TNF-α synthesis and inhibition of kallistatin expression through a ROS-JNK signaling pathway.

4. Kallistatin is a potent anti-inflammatory agent

Sepsis is a systemic inflammation in response to bacterial infection. Exogenous kallistatin attenuates inflammation and multiorgan damage in animals with cardiovascular and renal disorders [14, 17–20, 41]. For example, kallistatin gene delivery significantly reduces inflammatory responses and joint swelling in arthritic rats [19]. Kallistatin administration also suppresses inflammatory cell infiltration and prevents complement factor C5a-induced paw edema and vascular leakage in mice [20]. Local delivery of the kallistatin gene into rat heart enhances cardiac performance and attenuates inflammatory cell infiltration after acute myocardial ischemia/reperfusion (I/R) [41]. In salt-induced hypertensive rats, kallistatin therapy attenuates vascular and renal damage and reduces oxidative stress and inflammation [17, 18], while depletion of endogenous kallistatin augments organ injury and accentuates oxidative stress, inflammation, and fibrosis [47].

Kallistatin suppresses inflammatory responses by modulating differential signaling pathways. Kallistatin's active site is responsible for upregulating eNOS and SIRT1 expression, and thus increasing NO production [28]. NO, in turn, blocks TNF-α–induced ROS formation by inhibiting NADPH oxidase activity and NF-κB activation [58, 59]. Kallistatin via its active site induces the expression of SOCS3, a negative regulator of inflammation [48], thereby inhibiting LPS-induced TNF-α production in cultured macrophages [48, 60]. Moreover, kallistatin via its heparin-binding site antagonizes TNF-α–induced oxidative stress, NF-κB activation and inflammatory gene expression *in vitro* [20]. Likewise, kallistatin blocks HMGB1-mediated synthesis of inflammatory genes in endothelial cells [29]. Moreover, kallistatin ameliorates inflammation by blocking VEGF-induced endothelial cell permeability [16, 20]. Thus, kallistatin via its two structural domains exerts anti-inflammatory actions by: (1) stimulating eNOS and SIRT1 synthesis and NO formation; (2) increasing SOCS3 expression; (3) antagonizing TNF-α– and HMGB1-mediated inflammatory gene expression and oxidative stress; and (4) blocking VEGF-induced vascular permeability. Together, these findings indicate that kallistatin protects against organ damage by inhibiting inflammatory responses through multiple mechanisms.

5. Kallistatin attenuates organ damage and mortality in septic animal models

In Gram-negative infections, the cell wall component LPS (endotoxin) is the main initiator of the cascade of cellular reactions that lead to circulatory failure and organ injury [61]. *Staphylococcus aureus* is one of the most common Gram-positive bacteria isolated from patients with sepsis [61–63]. Gram-positive bacteria contain two major cell wall components, PepG and LTA, which cause sepsis and multiple organ injury in the absence of LPS [49–53]. A human kallistatin gene polymorphism is correlated with a decreased risk of developing acute kidney injury in patients with septic shock [64]. Kallistatin treatment exerts beneficial effects in Gram-negative and Gram-positive bacteremia, as well as "mixed" polymicrobial infection [29, 35, 48, 65]. Transgenic mice expressing kallistatin are highly resistant to mortality induced by LPS [66]. Moreover, kallistatin gene transfer reduces mortality, bacterial counts, and inflammatory cell numbers, as well as skin and liver damage, in a mouse model of streptococcal infection [65]. Kallistatin treatment in septic mice with polymicrobial infection attenuates lethality, peritoneal bacterial counts, renal injury and inflammation, and splenic apoptosis [29]. The protective effects of kallistatin in the kidney occurred in conjunction with reduced expression of TNF-α and HMGB1 and increased eNOS synthesis and NO levels [29]. NO inhibits oxidative organ damage by inactivating NAD(P)H oxidase activity [59]. Furthermore, delayed kallistatin administration after the onset of sepsis attenuates mortality, kidney and liver injury in mouse models of polymicrobial sepsis and endotoxemia [48]. Kallistatin treatment inhibits systemic inflammation by reducing circulatory levels of TNF-α and HMGB1, and dramatically upregulating SOCS3 expression in the kidney and lung [48]. Kallistatin delivery improves mortality, attenuates acute lung damage in LPS-induced septic mice, and inhibits ROS-mediated inflammation and apoptosis in cultured lung epithelial cells [35]. These findings indicate that kallistatin administration significantly enhances survival and protects against multiorgan damage during sepsis.

6. Kallistatin enhances bacterial killing by elevated oxidative stress

Oxidative stress has been shown to have beneficial effects with bacterial killing activity in inflammatory disorders [67, 68]. Human kallistatin treatment significantly enhances bacterial clearance and antimicrobial activity in group A streptococcus-infected mice by increasing superoxide production in immune cells [65]. Likewise, kallistatin administration leads to more than 10-fold decrease of bacterial counts in the peritoneal fluid of mice with polymirobial sepsis [29]. The bactericidal activity of kallistatin is most likely attributed to elevated ROS formation in peritoneal neutrophils [61]. Kallistatin also enhances immune cell viability and reduces their apoptosis [65]. Kallistatin through its active site increases SOCS3 expression in macrophages and SIRT1 synthesis in endothelial cells, but the effects are blocked by genistein [28]. Genistein also abolishes kallistatin's stimulation on endogenous H_2O_2 formation in vascular smooth muscle cells (unpublished results). These combined findings implicate a role of kallistatin's active site in enhancing ROS formation by interaction with a cell surface tyrosine kinase. Thus, kallistatin has a double-edged role in oxidative stress, depending on the pathological conditions. In addition to inhibiting oxidative stress and multiorgan damage, kallistatin is capable of exerting potent bactericidal activity by stimulating ROS formation in immune cells of animals with bacterial infection.

7. Signaling mechanisms mediated by kallistatin in sepsis

LPS (endotoxin) derived from Gram-negative bacteria, or PepG and LTA from Gram-positive bacteria, can lead to multiorgan injury and lethality by inducing the synthesis of TNF-α and HMGB1, thus elevating ROS formation [49–54]. TNF-α activates pro-inflammatory transcription factor NF-κB and the expression of inflammatory genes, such as ICAM-1 and VCAM-1. Kallistatin via its active site stimulates eNOS and SIRT1 expression and activation and increases NO formation in endothelial cells; NO in turn inhibits ROS formation [28, 59]. Kallistatin's active site is also crucial for increasing SOCS3 expression, leading to inhibition of LPS-induced TNF-α synthesis [48, 60]. Kallistatin via its heparin-binding domain blocks TNF-α– and HMGB1-induced NF-κB activation, inflammatory gene expression, and ROS formation [20, 29]. However, kallistatin's active site is involved in superoxide formation in immune cells, leading to a bacterial killing effect [65]. The signaling pathways mediated by kallistatin in the protection against sepsis are shown in **Figure 2**.

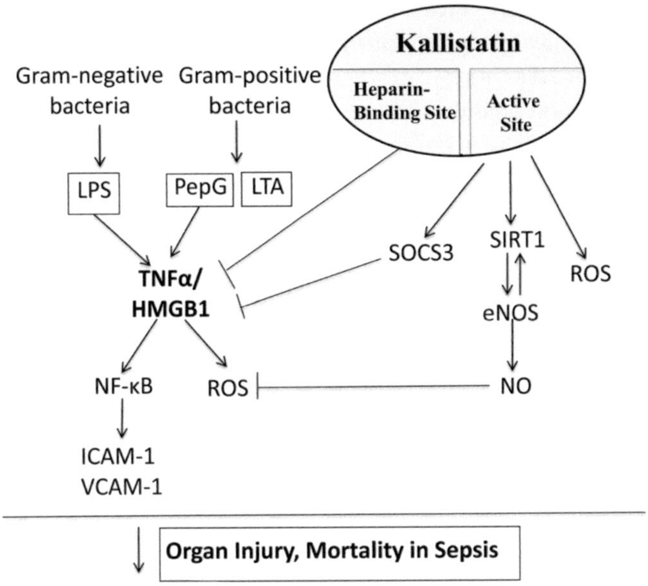

Figure 2. Signaling pathways mediated by kallistatin in sepsis. Kallistatin via its heparin-binding domain blocks TNF-α– and HMGB1-induced NF-κB activation, inflammatory gene expression, and ROS formation. Kallistatin via its active site stimulates eNOS, SIRT1 and SOCS3 expression, and NO formation, leading to inhibition of oxidative stress. Kallistatin increases ROS formation in immune cells. Kallistatin protects against organ injury and lethality during sepsis by modulating these differential signaling cascades.

8. Therapeutic implications of kallistatin

Sepsis is a systemic inflammatory response to infection. Kallistatin is an effective anti-inflammatory agent by triggering multiple signaling cascades in protection against septic shock. Reduction of plasma kallistatin levels is observed in patients with sepsis syndrome and is associated with severity of community-acquired pneumonia [33, 36]. Therefore, circulating kallistatin levels may serve as a biomarker for patients with severe sepsis and septic shock. Although the beneficial properties of kallistatin treatment in sepsis have been shown in animal studies, they still have yet to be confirmed in humans. Therapeutic application of kallistatin may provide a new approach for the treatment of sepsis and septic shock in humans.

http://dx.doi.org/10.5772/67988

9. Concluding remarks

Kallistatin levels are markedly reduced in septic shock and inflammatory disease. Kallistatin administration exerts beneficial effects during septic shock induced by Gram-negative bacteremia, Gram-positive bacteremia, or polymicrobial infection. Kallistatin possesses potent anti-inflammatory activities. Kallistatin via its two structural elements ameliorates inflammatory responses by regulating differential signaling cascades. Kallistatin's active site is crucial for stimulating eNOS, SIRT1, and SOCS3 expression and/or activation. Kallistatin via the heparin-binding site antagonizes both early (TNF-α) and late (HMGB1) cytokine-induced oxidative stress and inflammatory gene synthesis. Interestingly, kallistatin has a double-edged role in oxidative stress. In addition to suppressing oxidative stress, kallistatin exerts a marked bactericidal effect by stimulating ROS production in immune cells of mice with microbial infection. Kallistatin with its pleiotropic activities is an effective therapeutic agent in tissue injury and consequences of septic shock.

Acknowledgements

This work was supported by the National Institutes of Health grants HL118516 and HL 44083.

Author details

Julie Chao*, Pengfei Li and Lee Chao

*Address all correspondence to: chaoj@musc.edu

Department of Biochemistry, Molecular Biology, Medical University of South Carolina, Charleston, South Carolina, USA

References

[1] Gaieski DF, Edwards JM, Kallan MJ, Carr BG. Benchmarking the incidence and mortality of severe sepsis in the United States. Crit Care Med 2013; 41:1167-74.

[2] Angus DC, Linde-Zwirble WT, Lidicker J, Clermont G, Carcillo J, Pinsky MR. Epidemiology of severe sepsis in the United States: Analysis of incidence, outcome, and associated costs of care. Crit Care Med 2001; 29:1303-10.

[3] Vincent JL, Opal SM, Marshall JC, Tracey KJ. Sepsis definitions: Time for change. Lancet 2013; 381:774-5.

[4] Gogos CA, Drosou E, Bassaris HP, Skoutelis A. Pro- versus anti-inflammatory cytokine profile in patients with severe sepsis: A marker for prognosis and future therapeutic options. J Infect Dis 2000; 181:176-80.

[5] Reinhart K, Karzai W. Anti-tumor necrosis factor therapy in sepsis: Update on clinical trials and lessons learned. Crit Care Med 2001; 29:S121-5.

[6] Cohen J The immunopathogenesis of sepsis. Nature 2002; 420:885-91.

[7] Yoshimura A, Naka T, Kubo M. SOCS proteins, cytokine signalling and immune regulation. Nat Rev Immunol 2007; 7:454-65.

[8] Fang M, Dai H, Yu G, Gong F. Gene delivery of SOCS3 protects mice from lethal endotoxic shock. Cell Mol Immunol 2005; 2:373-7.

[9] Nair S, Pandey AD, Mukhopadhyay S. The PPE18 protein of Mycobacterium tuberculosis inhibits NF-kappaB/rel-mediated proinflammatory cytokine production by upregulating and phosphorylating suppressor of cytokine signaling 3 protein. J Immunol 2011; 186:5413-24.

[10] Riedemann NC, Guo RF, Ward PA. Novel strategies for the treatment of sepsis. Nat Med 2003; 9:517-24.

[11] Chao J, Chai KX, Chen LM, Xiong W, Chao S, Woodley-Miller C, Wang LX, Lu HS, Chao L. Tissue kallikrein-binding protein is a serpin. I. Purification, characterization, and distribution in normotensive and spontaneously hypertensive rats. J Biol Chem 1990; 265:16394-401.

[12] Chao J, Tillman DM, Wang MY, Margolius HS, Chao L. Identification of a new tissue-kallikrein-binding protein. Biochem J 1986; 239:325-31.

[13] Zhou GX, Chao L, Chao J. Kallistatin: A novel human tissue kallikrein inhibitor. Purification, characterization, and reactive center sequence. J Biol Chem 1992; 267: 25873-80.

[14] Gao L, Yin H, S Smith R Jr, Chao L, Chao J. Role of kallistatin in prevention of cardiac remodeling after chronic myocardial infarction. Lab Invest 2008; 88:1157-66.

[15] Miao RQ, Agata J, Chao L, Chao J. Kallistatin is a new inhibitor of angiogenesis and tumor growth. Blood 2002; 100:3245-52.

[16] Miao RQ, Chen V, Chao L, Chao J. Structural elements of kallistatin required for inhibition of angiogenesis. Am J Physiol Cell Physiol 2003; 284:C1604-13.

[17] Shen B, Gao L, Hsu YT, Bledsoe G, Hagiwara M, Chao L, Chao J. Kallistatin attenuates endothelial apoptosis through inhibition of oxidative stress and activation of Akt-eNOS signaling. Am J Physiol Heart Circ Physiol 2010; 299:H1419-27.

[18] Shen B, Hagiwara M, Yao YY, Chao L, Chao J. Salutary effect of kallistatin in salt-induced renal injury, inflammation, and fibrosis via antioxidative stress. Hypertension 2008; 51:1358-65.

[19] Wang CR, Chen SY, Wu CL, Liu MF, Jin YT, Chao L, Chao J. Prophylactic adenovirus-mediated human kallistatin gene therapy suppresses rat arthritis by inhibiting angiogenesis and inflammation. Arthritis Rheum 2005; 52:1319-24.

[20] Yin H, Gao L, Shen B, Chao L, Chao J. Kallistatin inhibits vascular inflammation by antagonizing tumor necrosis factor-alpha-induced nuclear factor kappaB activation. Hypertension 2010; 56:260-7.

[21] Chao J, Chao L. Biochemistry, regulation and potential function of kallistatin. Biol Chem Hoppe Seyler 1995; 376:705-13.

[22] Chen LM, Song Q, Chao L, Chao J. Cellular localization of tissue kallikrein and kallistatin mRNAs in human kidney. Kidney Int 1995; 48:690-7.

[23] Wolf WC, Harley RA, Sluce D, Chao L, Chao J. Localization and expression of tissue kallikrein and kallistatin in human blood vessels. J Histochem Cytochem 1999; 47:221-8.

[24] Chen VC, Chao L, Chao J. Reactive-site specificity of human kallistatin toward tissue kallikrein probed by site-directed mutagenesis. Biochim Biophys Acta 2000; 1479:237-46.

[25] Chen VC, Chao L, Chao J. Roles of the P1, P2, and P3 residues in determining inhibitory specificity of kallistatin toward human tissue kallikrein. J Biol Chem 2000; 275:38457-66.

[26] Chen VC, Chao L, Pimenta DC, Bledsoe G, Juliano L, Chao J. Identification of a major heparin-binding site in kallistatin. J Biol Chem 2001; 276:1276-84.

[27] Xiong W, Tang CQ, Zhou GX, Chao L, Chao J. In vivo catabolism of human kallikrein-binding protein and its complex with tissue kallikrein. J Lab Clin Med 1992; 119:514-21.

[28] Guo Y, Li P, Bledsoe G, Yang ZR, Chao L, Chao J. Kallistatin inhibits TGF-beta-induced endothelial-mesenchymal transition by differential regulation of microRNA-21 and eNOS expression. Exp Cell Res 2015; 337:103-10.

[29] Li P, Bledsoe G, Yang ZR, Fan H, Chao L, Chao J. Human kallistatin administration reduces organ injury and improves survival in a mouse model of polymicrobial sepsis. Immunology 2014; 142:216-26.

[30] Chao C, Madeddu P, Wang C, Liang Y, Chao L, Chao J. Differential regulation of kallikrein, kininogen, and kallikrein-binding protein in arterial hypertensive rats. Am J Physiol 1996; 271:F78-86.

[31] Chao J, Chen LM, Chai KX, Chao L. Expression of kallikrein-binding protein and alpha 1-antitrypsin genes in response to sex hormones, growth, inflammation and hypertension. Agents Actions Suppl 1992; 38 (Pt 1):174-81.

[32] Hatcher HC, Ma JX, Chao J, Chao L, Ottlecz A. Kallikrein-binding protein levels are reduced in the retinas of streptozotocin-induced diabetic rats. Invest Ophthalmol Vis Sci 1997; 38:658-64.

[33] Chao J, Schmaier A, Chen LM, Yang Z, Chao L. Kallistatin, a novel human tissue kallikrein inhibitor: Levels in body fluids, blood cells, and tissues in health and disease. J Lab Clin Med 1996; 127:612-20.

[34] Cheng Z, Lv Y, Pang S, Bai R, Wang M, Lin S, Xu T, Spalding D, Habib N, Xu R. Kallistatin, a new and reliable biomarker for the diagnosis of liver cirrhosis. Acta Pharm Sin B 2015; 5:194-200.

[35] Lin WC, Chen CW, Huang YW, Chao L, Chao J, Lin YS, Lin CF. Kallistatin protects against sepsis-related acute lung injury via inhibiting inflammation and apoptosis. Sci Rep 2015; 5:12463.

[36] Lin WC, Lu SL, Lin CF, Chen CW, Chao L, Chao J, Lin YS. Plasma kallistatin levels in patients with severe community-acquired pneumonia. Crit Care 2013; 17:R27.

[37] Stadnicki A, Mazurek U, Gonciarz M, Plewka D, Nowaczyk G, Orchel J, Pastucha E, Plewka A, Wilczok T, Colman RW. Immunolocalization and expression of kallistatin and tissue kallikrein in human inflammatory bowel disease. Dig Dis Sci 2003; 48:615-23.

[38] Ma JX, King LP, Yang Z, Crouch RK, Chao L, Chao J. Kallistatin in human ocular tissues: Reduced levels in vitreous fluids from patients with diabetic retinopathy. Curr Eye Res 1996; 15:1117-23.

[39] Chao J, Bledsoe G, Chao L. Protective role of kallistatin in vascular and organ injury. Hypertension 2016; 68:533-41.

[40] Zhu H, Chao J, Kotak I, Guo D, Parikh SJ, Bhagatwala J, Dong Y, Patel SY, Houk C, Chao L. Plasma kallistatin is associated with adiposity and cardiometabolic risk in apparently healthy African American adolescents. Metabolism 2013; 62:642-6.

[41] Chao J, Yin H, Yao YY, Shen B, Smith RS, Jr., Chao L. Novel role of kallistatin in protection against myocardial ischemia-reperfusion injury by preventing apoptosis and inflammation. Hum Gene Ther 2006; 17:1201-13.

[42] Zhang J, Yang Z, Li P, Bledsoe G, Chao L, Chao J. Kallistatin antagonizes Wnt/beta-catenin signaling and cancer cell motility via binding to low-density lipoprotein receptor-related protein 6. Mol Cell Biochem 2013; 379:295-301.

[43] Gao L, Li P, Zhang J, Hagiwara M, Shen B, Bledsoe G, Chang E, Chao L, Chao J. Novel role of kallistatin in vascular repair by promoting mobility, viability, and function of endothelial progenitor cells. J Am Heart Assoc 2014; 3:e001194.

[44] Li P, Guo Y, Bledsoe G, Yang Z, Chao L, Chao J. Kallistatin induces breast cancer cell apoptosis and autophagy by modulating Wnt signaling and microRNA synthesis. Exp Cell Res 2016; 340:305-14.

[45] Leu CH, Yang ML, Chung NH, Huang YJ, Su YC, Chen YC, Lin CC, Shieh GS, Chang MY, Wang SW, Chang Y, Chao J, Chao L, Wu CL, Shiau AL. Kallistatin ameliorates influenza virus pathogenesis by inhibition of kallikrein-related peptidase 1-mediated cleavage of viral hemagglutinin. Antimicrob Agents Chemother 2015; 59:5619-30.

[46] Shiau AL, Teo ML, Chen SY, Wang CR, Hsieh JL, Chang MY, Chang CJ, Chao J, Chao L, Wu CL, Lee CH. Inhibition of experimental lung metastasis by systemic lentiviral delivery of kallistatin. BMC Cancer 2010; 10:245.

[47] Liu Y, Bledsoe G, Hagiwara M, Shen B, Chao L, Chao J. Depletion of endogenous kallistatin exacerbates renal and cardiovascular oxidative stress, inflammation, and organ remodeling. Am J Physiol Renal Physiol 2012; 303:F1230-8.

[48] Li P, Guo Y, Bledsoe G, Yang ZR, Fan H, Chao L, Chao J. Kallistatin treatment attenuates lethality and organ injury in mouse models of established sepsis. Crit Care 2015; 19:200.

[49] Natanson C, Danner RL, Elin RJ, Hosseini JM, Peart KW, Banks SM, MacVittie TJ, Walker RI, Parrillo JE. Role of endotoxemia in cardiovascular dysfunction and mortality. *Escherichia coli* and *Staphylococcus aureus* challenges in a canine model of human septic shock. J Clin Invest 1989; 83:243-51.

[50] Wakabayashi G, Gelfand JA, Jung WK, Connolly RJ, Burke JF, Dinarello CA. Staphylococcus epidermidis induces complement activation, tumor necrosis factor and interleukin-1, a shock-like state and tissue injury in rabbits without endotoxemia. Comparison to *Escherichia coli*. J Clin Invest 1991; 87:1925-35.

[51] Mattsson E, Verhage L, Rollof J, Fleer A, Verhoef J, van Dijk H. Peptidoglycan and teichoic acid from *Staphylococcus epidermidis* stimulate human monocytes to release tumour necrosis factor-alpha, interleukin-1 beta and interleukin-6. FEMS Immunol Med Microbiol 1993; 7:281-7.

[52] Bhakdi S, Klonisch T, Nuber P, Fischer W. Stimulation of monokine production by lipoteichoic acids. Infect Immun 1991; 59:4614-20.

[53] Kengatharan KM, De Kimpe S, Robson C, Foster SJ, Thiemermann C. Mechanism of gram-positive shock: Identification of peptidoglycan and lipoteichoic acid moieties essential in the induction of nitric oxide synthase, shock, and multiple organ failure. J Exp Med 1998; 188:305-15.

[54] Mhatre MV, Potter JA, Lockwood CJ, Krikun G, Abrahams VM. Thrombin augments LPS-induced human endometrial endothelial cell inflammation via PAR1 activation. Am J Reprod Immunol 2016; 76:29-37.

[55] Khan SY, Awad EM, Oszwald A, Mayr M, Yin X, Waltenberger B, Stuppner H, Lipovac M, Uhrin P, Breuss JM. Premature senescence of endothelial cells upon chronic exposure to TNFalpha can be prevented by N-acetyl cysteine and plumericin. Sci Rep 2017; 7:39501.

[56] Ran X, Zhao W, Li W, Shi J, Chen X. Cryptotanshinone inhibits TNF-alpha-induced LOX-1 expression by suppressing reactive oxygen species (ROS) formation in endothelial cells. Korean J Physiol Pharmacol 2016; 20:347-55.

[57] Shen B, Chao L, Chao J. Pivotal role of JNK-dependent FOXO1 activation in downregulation of kallistatin expression by oxidative stress. Am J Physiol Heart Circ Physiol 2010; 298:H1048-54.

[58] Jiang MZ, Tsukahara H, Ohshima Y, Todoroki Y, Hiraoka M, Maeda M, Mayumi M. Effects of antioxidants and nitric oxide on TNF-alpha-induced adhesion molecule expression and NF-kappaB activation in human dermal microvascular endothelial cells. Life Sci 2004; 75:1159-70.

[59] Fujii H, Ichimori K, Hoshiai K, Nakazawa H. Nitric oxide inactivates NADPH oxidase in pig neutrophils by inhibiting its assembling process. J Biol Chem 1997; 272:32773-8.

[60] Dai Z, Lu L, Yang Z, Mao Y, Lu J, Li C, Qi W, Chen Y, Yao Y, Li L, Chen S, Zhang Y, Cai W, Yang X, Gao G. Kallikrein-binding protein inhibits LPS-induced TNF-alpha by upregulating SOCS3 expression. J Cell Biochem 2013; 114:1020-8.

[61] Wang JE, Dahle MK, McDonald M, Foster SJ, Aasen AO, Thiemermann C. Peptidoglycan and lipoteichoic acid in gram-positive bacterial sepsis: Receptors, signal transduction, biological effects, and synergism. Shock 2003; 20:402-14.

[62] Fluit AC, Jones ME, Schmitz FJ, Acar J, Gupta R, Verhoef J. Antimicrobial susceptibility and frequency of occurrence of clinical blood isolates in Europe from the SENTRY antimicrobial surveillance program, 1997 and 1998. Clin Infect Dis 2000; 30:454-60.

[63] Solomkin JS. Antibiotic resistance in postoperative infections. Crit Care Med 2001; 29:N97-9.

[64] Frank AJ, Sheu CC, Zhao Y, Chen F, Su L, Gong MN, Bajwa E, Thompson BT, Christiani DC. BCL2 genetic variants are associated with acute kidney injury in septic shock*. Crit Care Med 2012; 40:2116-23.

[65] Lu SL, Tsai CY, Luo YH, Kuo CF, Lin WC, Chang YT, Wu JJ, Chuang WJ, Liu CC, Chao L, Chao J, Lin YS. Kallistatin modulates immune cells and confers anti-inflammatory response to protect mice from group A streptococcal infection. Antimicrob Agents Chemother 2013; 57:5366-72.

[66] Chen LM, Chao L, Chao J. Beneficial effects of kallikrein-binding protein in transgenic mice during endotoxic shock. Life Sci 1997; 60:1431-5.

[67] Miller RA, Britigan BE. Role of oxidants in microbial pathophysiology. Clin Microbiol Rev 1997; 10:1-18.

[68] Lukaszewicz AC, Gontier G, Faivre V, Ouanounou I, Payen D. Elevated production of radical oxygen species by polymorphonuclear neutrophils in cerebrospinal fluid infection. Ann Intensive Care 2012; 2:10.

Section 4

Dietry Fatty Acids and Sepsis

Chapter 4

The Role of Fish Oil Feeding Rich in ω-3 Polyunsaturated Fatty Acids in Patients with Sepsis and Septic Shock

Vasilios Papaioannou

Additional information is available at the end of the chapter

http://dx.doi.org/10.5772/68041

Abstract

Different clinical studies have demonstrated that fish oil, rich in the very-long-chain ω-3 polyunsaturated fatty acids (PUFAs), has immunomodulatory effects, suppressing the production of pro-inflammatory cytokines in diverse groups of critically ill patients. Moreover, such compounds have been found to attenuate the inflammatory response within 2–3 days upon parenteral administration. Recent experimental data suggest that activation of the cholinergic anti-inflammatory pathway constitutes a novel mechanism of such immune-regulatory effects. Since enhanced vagal tone has been associated with decreased cytokine secretion, novel monitoring tools of its activity at the bedside are needed, in order to evaluate nutritional manipulation of inflammatory response in the critically ill. The present chapter provides an overview of the mechanisms of action through which ω-3 PUFA modulates immune response in critically ill patients suffering from sepsis and septic shock. Furthermore, it summarizes the current evidence regarding clinical effects from administration of fish oil rich in ω-3 PUFAs in septic patients. Finally, it presents data that suggest the existence of a continuous interrelation between immune status and autonomic nervous system during systemic inflammation and proposes novel tools of autonomic nervous system monitoring at the bedside, in order to assess pharmacological manipulation of immune response by ω-3 PUFAs in acute illness.

Keywords: ω-3 fatty acids, lipid emulsions, sepsis, heart rate variability, enteral, parenteral, nutrition, critical care, autonomic nervous system

INTECH
open science | open minds

© 2017 The Author(s). Licensee InTech. This chapter is distributed under the terms of the Creative Commons Attribution License (http://creativecommons.org/licenses/by/3.0), which permits unrestricted use, distribution, and reproduction in any medium, provided the original work is properly cited. (cc) BY

1. Introduction

Acute systemic inflammation is the host response to various insults, such as infection, trauma, hemorrhage, etc., and is mediated by the release in circulation of different cytokines, such as tumor necrosis factor alpha (TNF-α) and interleukin-1 (IL-1), IL-4, IL-6, or IL-10 [1, 2]. Such mediators possess both pro- and anti-inflammatory properties. Furthermore, they are capable to activate the hypothalamo-pituitary-adrenal (HPA) axis and both the sympathetic and parasympathetic divisions of the autonomic nervous system (ANS), which subsequently may affect the immune response [1].

However, safety mechanisms do sometimes fail, leading to a new continuum of disease—sepsis, septic shock, and multiple organ dysfunction syndrome (MODS). In this respect, patients develop nutrient deficiencies, which are associated with an increased risk of developing infections, organ failure, and death [3]. Consequently, artificial nutrition via the enteral or parenteral route is considered as an integral part of standard care. Recently, the concept of pharmaconutrition has emerged as an alternative approach, considering nutrition an active therapy rather than an adjunctive care [4]. Thus, specific nutrients have been designed to modulate the host immune response and suppress systemic inflammation. Moreover, lipid components of parenteral nutrition have been found to provide powerful bioactive molecules that may act to reduce inflammatory responses [5].

Different clinical trials have shown that fatty acids from fish oil can be considered as powerful disease-modifying nutrients in patients with acute lung injury and sepsis [6, 7]. Particularly, feeding with fish oil rich in the very-long-chain, ω-3 polyunsaturated fatty acids (PUFAs), eicosapentaenoic acid (EPA), and docasahexaenoic acid (DHA) has been found to attenuate the production of different cytokines, chemokines, and other effectors of innate immune response [8]. In addition, the recent discovery of resolvins generated by EPA and DHA has shed more light on resolution of inflammation, as a possible mechanism of the anti-inflammatory actions of ω-3 PUFAs during systemic inflammation [9]. However, oral administration of these compounds is required for several weeks to affect metabolic and inflammatory pathways in humans. Nevertheless, it has been recently demonstrated that intravenous administration of fat emulsions rich in ω-3 PUFAs can lead to their rapid incorporation into phospholipids of different cells, such as platelets or monocytes, within the first 2 days of feeding, reducing serum pro-inflammatory cytokines over the next 7–8 days [10–12]. This may affect membrane fluidity, ion channel opening, or different signal pathways, leading to decreased production of TNF-α and IL-6 [8, 10]. The bypass of the intestinal process of absorption that is significantly delayed during critical illness could be another reason for such immediate effects.

2. Anti-inflammatory mechanisms of ω-3 PUFA

There are two types of naturally occurring essential fatty acids (EFAs) which cannot be synthesized in the body and need to be obtained in our diet, the ω-6 series derived from linoleic acid (LA) and the ω-3 series derived from α-linolenic acid (ALA). Both the ω-6 and ω-3

http://dx.doi.org/10.5772/68041

series are metabolized by the same set of enzymes to their responsive long-chain metabolites. In general, the term EFA includes all unsaturated fatty acids. In this respect, all EFAs are PUFAs, but all PUFAs are not EFAs [13]. The major metabolic pathways of ω-3 include (1) incorporation into triglycerides that are found in circulating lipoproteins; (2) incorporation into phospholipids of either circulating lipoproteins as well or part of cellular membranes; (3) be circulated as free (nonesterified) fatty acids (FFAs) in the plasma, mostly bound in albumin; and (4) undergo oxidation generating substrates for ATP synthesis. ω-3 PUFAs incorporated in membrane phospholipids are capable to affect membrane fluidity and membrane-associated protein function. Furthermore, they can be cleaved by different phospholipases, giving rise to FFAs that subsequently are further oxidized to form various metabolites that are called eicosanoids (such as prostaglandins and leukotrienes) [8, 13]. These eicosanoids derived from EPA through different cyclo- and lipo-oxygenases are generally considered less pro-inflammatory in relation with their counterparts derived from the very-long-chain ω-6 PUFA, such as arachidonic acid (AA). The major PUFA-derived mediators are lipoxins, resolvins, and protectins which are highly active and are involved in different physiological and pathophysiological processes. In this respect, experimental studies have shown that protectin D1 (PD1) reduces inflammatory infiltration, enhances phagocytosis of apoptotic neutrophils by macrophages, and, finally, increases macrophage migration to sites of antigen presentation. As a result, these metabolites seem to both inhibit the initiation of an overwhelmed inflammatory response and accelerate at the same time its resolution [8, 13].

The ω-3 PUFA can also inhibit the activity of nuclear factor kB (NF-kB), which is considered a pivotal pro-inflammatory transcription factor and induces the expression of many pro-inflammatory genes, mediating through the production of different cytokines, the innate immune response [8, 9].

3. ω-3 PUFA, the autonomic nervous system, and heart rate variability

Different experimental studies have confirmed that there is a continuous cross talk between the brain and the immune response to different inflammatory insults during both an acute and chronic inflammation. In this respect, it has been postulated that the brain may coordinate and affect at the same time the immune response. The first mechanism is based on the activation of vagus nerve afferent fibers, which convey the information that an inflammatory response takes place, through different mediators, such as cytokines [14–16].

Cytokines can activate visceral vagus afferent fibers which terminate within the dorsal vagal complex (DVC) of the medulla oblongata. The nucleus tractus solitarius (NTS) and the dorsal motor nucleus (DMN) of the vagus are part of DVC and give projections to hypothalamic paraventricular nucleus (PVN) that is responsible for the synthesis and release of corticotropin-releasing hormone (CRH), with subsequent production of adrenocorticotropin hormone (ACTH) from the anterior pituitary. ACTH is the main inducer of the synthesis of immunosuppressive glucocorticoids from the adrenal cortex. DMN that is connected with NTS is believed to constitute the main site of origin of preganglionic vagus efferent fibers. NTS is also connected to rostral ventrolateral medulla (RVLM), which increases noradrenergic preganglionic neurons' depolarization in the spinal cord [17]. In conclusion, the brain may alter the immune response through the activation of both the sympathetic (SNS) and parasympathetic nervous systems (PNS), as well as the activation of the HPA axis. In this respect, the SNS may induce local inflammatory response through α_2-subtype adrenoreceptor stimulation by norepinephrine (NE), in the early stage of inflammation. Nevertheless, stimulation of β_2-subtype adrenoreceptor-cAMP-protein kinase A pathway can also reduce pro-inflammatory cytokine production [18–20], suggesting that SNS activation can both protect the organism from the detrimental effects of pro-inflammatory cytokines and increase at same time local inflammatory response [21, 22].

Apart from the SNS, a link between the PNS of the ANS and immunoregulatory processes has been suggested. Thus, acetylcholine is capable to decrease TNF-α production from human macrophage cultures and immune cells located in the spleen upon stimulation with endotoxin, leading to its reduced release into the circulation. This effect is mediated by the specific α7-subunit of the nicotinic acetylcholine receptor [23–25]. Acetylcholine is also effective in suppressing other pro-inflammatory cytokines such as IL-1β, IL-6, and high mobility group box 1 (HMGB1) [26].

A novel anti-inflammatory mechanism of lipid-diet immunosuppressive effects has been recently described by Luyer and colleagues [27]. They demonstrated that high-fat enteral nutrition was able to lead to attenuation of systemic inflammation in rats subjected to hemorrhagic shock, through stimulation of cholecystokinin (CCK) receptors and subsequent activation of the cholinergic anti-inflammatory pathway.

In this respect, Tracey has suggested that for the development of new monitoring tools of the ω-3 PUFA effects upon the cholinergic pathway in the clinic, new surrogate markers are needed [28], such as heart rate variability (HRV) analysis that is the variability of R-R series in the electrocardiogram (ECG). HRV reflects both sympathetic and parasympathetic inputs upon the heart and can be estimated via frequency domain methods, which calculate the different frequency components of a heart rate signal through a fast Fourier transformation (FFT) of an R-R time series [29]. The method displays in a plot at least three peaks—fast periodicities [high frequency (HF), 0.15–0.4 Hz] which are largely due to the influence of vagal tone—and has the largest impact on HRV. Recently, it has been found that central muscarinic cholinergic stimulation (usually in the context of balancing cytokine production) is also accompanied by activation of the HF component of HRV and an instantaneous increase in total variability [30]. Low-frequency periodicities (LF, 0.04–0.15 Hz) are produced by baroreflex feedback loops, affected mostly by sympathetic modulation of the heart, and very low frequency (VLF) periodicities (less than 0.04 Hz) are related to vasomotor activity. The LF/HF ratio has been considered as a surrogate marker of sympathovagal balance [29, 31].

Studying physiological signals of critically ill patients can easily identify "hidden" information, which can estimate variability and information content (entropy) as a measure of complexity, within time series [32]. It has been suggested that such measures are significantly altered during critical illness and may predict different outcomes of interest, such as the onset of septic shock and late organ dysfunction [33]. In addition, implementation of variability analysis of physiological signals at the bedside might give rise to new markers of disease. Such "physiomarkers" are generally considered more appropriate for better and more accurate early warning signs for patients, since they can be easily measured at the bedside. On the contrary, it has been repeatedly demonstrated that various "biomarkers" such as cytokines

http://dx.doi.org/10.5772/68041

exhibit marked interdependence, pleiotropy (multiple effects), and redundancy (multiple cytokines with the same effect). At the same time, their plasma concentrations fluctuate from day to day and correlate poorly with classic physiologic variables in septic patients [33, 34].

Both LF and HF frequency components and overall HRV are significantly reduced in septic patients, whereas the degree of attenuation has been found to be prognostic of survival [22, 35]. The reduction in instantaneous HRV has been associated with an overproduction of cytokines [36], whereas pharmacological stimulation of the efferent vagus nerve has been found to increase the HF component of HRV and inhibit at the same time TNF-α secretion in septic animals [37]. Many studies have shown that oral supplementation of ω-3 PUFAs increases instantaneous HRV, reduces LF/HF ratio, and confers protection against ischemia-induced ventricular tachycardia and sudden cardiac death [38, 39]. In this respect, Christensen and colleagues [39] demonstrated that fish oil feeding can induce an incorporation of DHA into the membranes of granulocytes that is associated with a dose-response increase in HRV and may protect against serious ventricular arrhythmias. In a recent study [40], the intravenous administration of fish oil with ω-3 PUFAs, before endotoxin injection in healthy volunteers, was able to blunt fever response and sympathetic stimulation and enhance vagal tone, estimated with HRV analysis. This reduction was associated with a significant decrease in plasma norepinephrine and adrenocorticotropin hormone (ACTH) levels. Such effects of fish oil reflect an enhanced efferent vagal activity via a central-acting mechanism due to a possible suppression of pro-inflammatory cytokines, which have been found to inhibit central vagal neurons [8, 41].

However, different interventional studies on ω-3 PUFAs and HRV in patients with heart disease have found inconsistent results, with only 8 out of the 20 trials published so far, supporting a beneficial effect on HRV [42]. Thus, Mozaffarian et al. [43] found that individuals with the highest fish consumption (≥5 meals/week) exhibited 1.5 ms greater HRV than those with the lowest fish consumption. Moreover, this modest reduction in HRV was associated with only a 1.1% reduction in the relative risk for sudden cardiac death. As we have stated elsewhere [44], "reasons for such inconsistency might include heterogeneous populations, limited sample sizes or different study protocols with variable administered doses of ω-3 PUFA and length of intervention." Furthermore, "different methods of measurement of HRV with variable time of recordings could be an additional confounder" [42–44]. Another potential limitation of such measures could be associated with the fact that a reduction in pacemaker funny current rather than an alteration in autonomic neural output was found to be responsible for heart rate reduction and increase in HRV in an animal study with administration of ω-3 PUFAs [45]. Nevertheless, a potential impact of autonomic tone on HRV cannot be evaluated in this study since experiments were performed in denervated hearts.

In conclusion, an association has been suggested between increased HRV and fish oil administration in different groups of patients with cardiovascular diseases [38, 39, 42]. However, the possible relationship between HRV changes and inflammatory markers during fish oil feeding has not been studied yet, in septic patients. Thus, we think that a promising approach could be the assessment of the relationship between vagal activity estimated with HRV and inflammatory markers in septic patients, during parenteral fish oil feeding. In this case, we assume a beneficial effect of ω-3 PUFAs on HRV and cytokine response, early in the course of disease.

4. Clinical studies

In Europe there are currently three available lipid emulsions containing ω-3 fish oil for IV administration: Omegaven (Fresenius Kabi, Germany) that is a 10% fish oil emulsion supplement; Lipoplus/Lipidem (B Braun, Germany) that contains a mixture of 50% medium-chain triglycerides (MCT) and 40% soybean oil (SO) that is rich in ω-6 PUFA, such as LA and 10% fish oil; and Smoflipid (Fresenius Kabi, Germany) that is a four-oil mixture of 30% soybean oil, 30% MCT, 25% olive oil, and 15% fish oil [13].

Numerous studies in critically ill patients have found favorable effects of ω-3 fish oil on different aspects of inflammatory response. Mayer and colleagues [10] randomized 21 septic patients requiring parenteral nutrition to receive an IV lipid emulsion rich either in ω-3 (Omegaven) or ω-6 (Lipoven) PUFAs. They were able to show that the first group within 2 days of infusion demonstrated a rapid incorporation of ω-3 fatty acids into mononuclear leukocyte membranes. In addition, fish oil rich in ω-3 was found to suppress generation of pro-inflammatory cytokines from mononuclear leukocytes upon ex vivo stimulation with endotoxin. Heller and colleagues [46] demonstrated that IV ω-3 PUFA administration (Omegaven) in 661 surgical critically ill patients improved survival and reduced infection rates, antibiotic requirement, and length of stay in a dose-dependent manner. Moreover, IV fish oil was found safe, conferring significant clinical benefits when administered in doses between 0.1 and 0.2 gr/Kg/day. In two other studies evaluating fish oil parenteral administration in surgical patients admitted to the Intensive Care Unit (ICU), it was found that although a short-term (<5 days) administration influences immune parameters, postoperative administration may further reduce length of stay and infectious complications in the ICU [12, 47]. In this respect Braga et al. concluded that ω-3 should be given prior to surgery in order to enhance their anti-inflammatory effects in the postoperative period [48].

Barbosa et al. [11] evaluated the effects of IV fish oil administration (Lipoplus) for 5 days in 25 septic ICU patients. They found a significant decrease in IL-6 plasma concentration, reduced hospital length of stay and amelioration in gas exchange during the sixth day of stay in the ICU.

In 2014, Manzanares and colleagues [49] after aggregating six randomized controlled trials (RCTs) evaluating the effects of parenteral fish oil on relevant clinical outcomes in a heterogeneous group of critically ill patients were able to demonstrate a significant reduction in mortality and duration of mechanical ventilation. In 2015, the same group of researchers, after analyzing data from 10 RCTs involving 733 patients, was not able to find any survival benefit from parenteral fish oil feeding in septic patients [50]. Nevertheless, a reduction in the incidence of infections and a trend toward reduced duration of mechanical ventilation and length of stay in ICU were reported. Furthermore, intravenous fish oil feeding exhibited a nonsignificant trend toward reduced mortality. Since conflicting data have been originated from other systematic reviews and meta-analyses [51, 52] "low sample size and heterogeneity of the cohorts included do not permit a final recommendation on the use of ω-3 PUFAs as a pharmaconutrient strategy in septic ICU patients" [50].

The European Society for Clinical Nutrition and Metabolism (ESPEN) Guidelines on Parenteral Nutrition in Intensive Care has suggested that both EPA and DHA can affect cell membranes and, subsequently, reduce the intensity of inflammatory response. As a result, fish oil-enriched lipid emulsions might decrease duration of hospitalization in critically ill patients [53]. Canadian recommendations also endorse the use of fish oil-enriched lipid emulsions when parenteral nutrition is indicated [54]. Finally, the American Society for Parenteral and Enteral Nutrition (ASPEN) in its recently published guidelines cannot recommend fish oil parenteral feeding in critically ill patients at this time, due to lack of availability on the market of these products in the United States, despite approval by the FDA in 2013 [55]. Nevertheless, it considers as appropriate its future administration either in patients with septic shock who are candidates for parenteral nutrition due to hemodynamic compromise, such as hypotensive (mean arterial blood pressure < 50 mm Hg); patients for whom catecholamine agents (e.g. norepinephrine, epinephrine) are being initiated and patients for whom escalating doses are required to maintain hemodynamic stability; or surgical postoperative patients who are not eligible for enteral nutrition (e.g. short bowel) [55].

Different studies have also assessed potential differences between SO and fish oil lipid IV fat emulsions in septic patients. In a recent systematic review of 12 RCTS including 806 patients by Manzanares and colleagues, no significant difference in outcome benefits was found [56]. In another meta-analysis of eight RCTS involving 391 patients by Palmer et al. [52], a significant reduction in hospital length of stay was demonstrated by nearly 10 days in those receiving ω-3 fish oil in relation with either SO-based or SO + MCT-based lipid emulsions. However, no differences were seen between groups with regard to ICU length of stay, infectious complications, and mortality. The strongest evidence in favor of fish oil PUFAs than SO-based lipid emulsions comes from small observational studies [55]. In this respect, data collected from an International Nutritional Survey showed a significantly lower ICU length of stay, reduced duration of mechanical ventilation, and reduced ICU mortality in septic patients receiving fish oil PUFAs when compared with SO-based lipid emulsions [57].

Another issue that has been tested in different RCTs is associated with safety and tolerability. Recently, a meta-analysis of 23 trials involving 1503 patients receiving long-term parenteral nutrition with IV fish oil found no evidence of any deleterious effects [58]. Consequently, ESPEN Guidelines on Parenteral Nutrition in Intensive Care suggests that lipids and essential fatty acids should be an integral part of the regimen to provide energy and should be administered at a rate of 0.7–1.5 gr/Kg over 12–24 h [53].

Considering enteral administration of lipid emulsions rich in ω-3 PUFAs in critically ill patients with sepsis and septic shock, strong evidence is still lacking. While early studies and meta-analyses suggested reduced infection rates, ICU length of stay, and duration of mechanical ventilation, in both medical and surgical patients in a general ICU [59], Heyland and colleagues found a modest reduction in hospital length of stay, particularly in medical patients [60]. Furthermore and according to ASPEN Guidelines, current evidence does not support the use of enteral fish oil administration, particularly in medical ICU patients, due to heterogeneity of studies, variety of experimental and commercial lipid formulations, variable dosage of individual components, and increased costs [55]. Finally, two recent meta-analyses showed that the effect of fish oil lipid emulsions on mortality in septic patients was not influenced by the route of administration (enteral vs. parenteral) [50, 61].

5. Conclusions

Many experimental studies have confirmed that ω-3 PUFAs possess different anti-inflammatory properties. Either through effect on membrane fluidity with subsequent attenuation of cytokine production or through indirect activation of the cholinergic anti-inflammatory pathway (immunoreflex), fish oil lipids have demonstrated immune-regulatory activities in different experimental settings. As a result, different investigators have evaluated their role in different groups of patients exhibiting systemic inflammation, such as surgical or septic patients treated in the ICU. However, extreme heterogeneity in patients' populations, route of administration, doses and duration of therapy, as well as commercially available products limits generalizability of results derived from numerous systematic reviews and meta-analyses. Consequently and since the current evidence is still too weak and sparse to make recommendations about the role of fish oil in the treatment of the critically ill, we suggest that HRV could be adopted as end point for monitoring nutritional manipulation of inflammatory response at the bedside, helping translation of basic science results into successful randomized controlled trials. In this case, we assume that ω-3 PUFAs upon parenteral administration will be rapidly incorporated into the phospholipid membranes of different immune cell types, reducing the inflammatory response and increasing HRV.

In this respect, 24 h recordings and longitudinal changes of HRV in two groups of septic patients with similar severity of disease and receiving parenteral nutrition with the same volume of glucose, nitrogen, and fat but different lipid composition could be tested. In the case that HRV metrics predict outcomes of interest, such as lower infection rate and/or attenuated organ dysfunction, such a study might identify a unique value of HRV analysis as a monitoring tool of inflammatory modulation by fish oil feeding, in septic patients. Another potential use of HRV in artificial nutrition of septic patients as has been suggested by Tracey [62] could be its adoption as a physiomarker to early identify patients with reduced vagal tone. In this case, a susceptibility to increased inflammation can be assumed, whereas HRV metrics might serve as an early alarm to identify patients who might benefit from pharmacological stimulation of the cholinergic anti-inflammatory pathway, such as ω-3 PUFAs [62].

Author details

Vasilios Papaioannou

Address all correspondence to: vapapa@med.duth.gr

Democritus University of Thrace, School of Medicine, Alexandroupolis Hospital, ICU, Alexandroupolis, Greece

References

[1] Koj A. Initiation of acute phase response and synthesis of cytokines. Biochim Biophys Acta 1997; 1317: 84-94.

[2] Webster JI, Tonelli L, Sternberg EM. Neuroendocrine regulation of immunity. Annu Rev Immunol 2002; 20: 125-163.

[3] Goode HF, Cowley HC, Walker BE, et al. Decreased antioxidant status and increased lipid peroxidation in patients with septic shock and secondary organ dysfunction. Crit Care Med 1995; 23: 646-651.

[4] Jones NE, Heyland DK. Pharmaconutrition: a new emerging paradigm. Curr Opin Gastroenterol 2008; 24: 215-222.

[5] Wanten GJ, Calder PC. Immune modulation by parenteral lipid emulsions. Am J Clin Nutr 2007; 85: 1171-1184.

[6] Singer P, Theilla M, Fisher H, et al. Benefit of an enteral diet enriched with eicosapentaenoic acid and gamma-linolenic acid in ventilated patients with acute lung injury. Crit Care Med 2006; 34: 1033-1038.

[7] Pontes-Arruda A, Aragao AM, Albuquerque JD. Effects of enteral feeding with eicosapentaenoic acid, gamma-linolenic acid, and antioxidants in mechanically ventilated patients with severe sepsis and septic shock. Crit Care Med 2006; 34: 2325-2333.

[8] Singer P, Shapiro H, Theilla M, et al. Anti-inflammatory properties of omega-3 fatty acids in critical illness: novel mechanisms and an integrative perspective. Intensive Care Med 2008; 34: 1580-1592.

[9] Serhan CN, Savill J. Resolution of inflammation: the beginning programs the end. Nat Immunol 2005; 6: 1191-1197.

[10] Mayer K, Gokorsch S, Fegbeutel C, et al. Parenteral nutrition with fish oil modulates cytokine response in patients with sepsis. Am J Respir Crit Care Med 2003; 167: 1321-1328.

[11] Barbosa VM, Miles EA, Calhau C, et al. Effects of a fish oil containing lipid emulsion on plasma phospholipid fatty acids, inflammatory markers, and clinical outcomes in septic patients: a randomized, controlled clinical trial. Crit Care 2010; 14: R5.

[12] Han YY, Lai SL, Ko WJ, et al. Effects of fish oil on inflammatory modulation in surgical intensive care unit patients. Nutr Clin Pract 2012; 27: 91-98.

[13] Klek S. Omega-3 fatty acids in modern parenteral nutrition: a review of the current evidence. J Clin Med 2016; 5: 34, doi: 10.3390/jcm5030034.

[14] Kumar V, Sharma A. Is immunomodulation a future therapeutic approach for sepsis? Int Immunopharmacol 2010; 10(1): 9-17.

[15] Berthhoud HR, Neuhuber WL. Functional anatomy of afferent vagal system. Auton Neurosci 2000; 85: 1-17.

[16] Tracey KJ. The inflammatory reflex. Nature 2002; 420: 853-859.

[17] Tracey KJ. Physiology and immunology of the cholinergic anti-inflammatory pathway. J Clin Invest 2007; 117: 289-296.

[18] Elenkov IJ, Wilder RL, Chrousos GP, et al. The sympathetic nerve-an integrative interface between two supersystems: the brain and the immune system. Pharmacol Rev 2000; 52: 595-638.

[19] Zhou M, Yang S, Koo DJ, et al. The role of Kupffer cell α_2 adrenoceptors in norepinephrine-induced TNF-α production. Biochim Biophys Acta 2001; 1537: 49-57.

[20] van der Poll T, Coyle SM, Barbosa K, et al. Epinephrine inhibits tumor necrosis factor-α and potentiates interleukin-10 production during human endotoxemia. J Clin Invest 1996; 97: 713-719.

[21] Chrousos GP. The hypothalamic-pituitary-adrenal axis and immune-mediated inflammation. New Engl J Med 1995; 332(20): 1351-1362.

[22] Papaioannou V, Dragoumanis C, Theodorou V, et al. Relation of heart rate variability to serum levels of C-reactive protein, interleukin 6 and 10 in patients with sepsis and septic shock. J Crit Care 2009; 24: 625.e1-625.e7.

[23] Wang H, Yu M, Ochani M, et al. Nicotinic acetylcholine receptor α7 subunit is an essential regulator of inflammation. Nature 2003; 421: 384-388.

[24] Pavlov VA, Wang H, Czura CJ, et al. The cholinergic anti-inflammatory pathway: a missing link in neuroimmunomodulation. Mol Med 2003; 9(5-8): 125-134.

[25] Huston JM, Ochani M, Rossas-Ballina M, et al. Splenectomy inactivates the cholinergic anti-inflammatory pathway during lethal endotoxemia and polymicrobial sepsis. J Exp Med 2006; 203: 1623-1628.

[26] Wang H, Liao H, Ochani M, et al. Cholinergic agonists inhibit HMGB1 release and improve survival in experimental sepsis. Nat Med 2004; 10: 1216-1221.

[27] Luyer MD, Greve JWM, Hadfoune M, et al. Nutritional stimulation of cholecystokinin receptors inhibits inflammation via the vagus nerve. J Exp Med 2005; 202: 1023-1029.

[28] Tracey KJ. Fat meets the cholinergic anti-inflammatory pathway. J Exp Med 2005; 202: 1017-1021.

[29] Task Force of the European Society of Cardiology and the North American Society of Pacing and Electrophysiology. Standards of measurement, physiological interpretation and clinical use. Circulation 1996; 93: 1043-1065.

[30] Munfold RS, Tracey KJ. Is severe sepsis a neuroendocrine disease? J Mol Med 2002; 8(8): 437-442.

[31] Malik M, Camm AJ. Components of heart rate variability: what they really mean and what we really measure. Am J Cardiol 1993; 72: 821-822.

[32] Kennedy H. Heart rate variability-a potential, noninvasive prognostic index in the critically ill patient. Crit Care Med 1998; 26: 213-214.

[33] Seely AJE, Christou NV. Multiple organ dysfunction syndrome: exploring the paradigm of complex nonlinear systems. Crit Care Med 2000; 28: 2193-2200.

[34] Friedland JS, Porter JC, Daryanani S, et al. Plasma proinflammatory cytokine concentrations, APACHE III scores and survival in patients in an intensive care unit. Crit Care Med 1996; 24: 1775-1781.

[35] Schmidt H, Muller-Werdan U, Hoffmann T, et al. Autonomic dysfunction predicts mortality in patients with multiple organ dysfunction syndrome of different age groups. Crit Care Med 2005; 33: 1994-2002.

[36] Tateishi Y, Oda S, Nakamura M, et al. Depressed heart rate variability is associated with high IL-6 blood level and decline in blood pressure in septic patients. Shock 2007; 28(5): 549-553.

[37] Pavlov VA, Ochani M, Gallowitsch-Puerta M, et al. Central muscarinic cholinergic regulation of the systemic inflammatory response during endotoxemia. Proc Natl Acad Sci USA 2006; 103: 5219-5223.

[38] Abuissa H, O' Keefe JH, Harris Jr W, et al. Autonomic function, omega-3, and cardiovascular risk. Chest 2005; 127: 1088-1091.

[39] Christensen JH, Christensen MS, Dyerberg J, et al. Heart rate variability and fatty acid content of blood cell membranes: a dose-response study with n-3 fatty acids. Am J Clin Nutr 1999; 70: 331-337.

[40] Pluess T-T, Hayoz D, Berger MM, et al. Intravenous fish oil blunts the physiological response to endotoxin in healthy subjects. Intensive Care Med 2007; 33: 789-797.

[41] Das UN. Beneficial effects of n-3 fatty acids in cardiovascular diseases: but, why and how? Prostaglandins Leukot Essent Fatty Acids 2000; 63: 351-362.

[42] Christensen JH. Omega-3 polyunsaturated fatty acids and heart rate variability. Front Physiol 2011; 2: 84, doi: 10.3389/fphys.2011.00084.

[43] Mozaffarian D, Stein PK, Prineas RJ, et al. Dietary fish ω-3 fatty acid consumption and heart rate variability in US adults. Circulation 2008; 117: 1130-1137.

[44] Papaioannou V, Pneumatikos I, Maglaveras N. Association of heart rate variability and inflammatory response in patients with cardiovascular diseases: current strengths and limitations. Front Physiol 2013; 4 (174): 1-13.

[45] Verkerk AO, den Ruijiter HM, Bourier J, et al. Dietary fish oil reduces pacemaker current and heart rate in rabbit. Heart Rhythm 2009; 6: 1485-1492.

[46] Heller AR, Rossler S, Litz RJ, et al. Omega-3 fatty acids improve the diagnosis-related clinical outcome. Crit Care Med 2006; 34: 972-979.

[47] De Miranda Torrinhas RS, Santana R, Garcia T, et al. Parenteral fish oil as a pharmacological agent to modulate post-operative immune response: a randomized double-blind and controlled clinical trial in patients with gastrointestinal cancer. Clin Nutr 2013; 32: 503-510.

[48] Braga M, Wischmeyer D, Drover J, et al. Clinical evidence for pharmaconutrition in major elective surgery. J Parenter Enteral Nutr 2013; 37: 66S–72S.

[49] Manzanares W, Dhaliwal R, Jurewitsch B, et al. Parenteral fish oil lipid emulsions in the critically ill: a systematic review and meta-analysis. JPEN J Parenter Enteral Nutr 2014; 38: 20-28.

[50] Manzanares W, Langlois PL, Dhaliwal R, et al. Intravenous fish oil lipid emulsions: an updated systematic review and meta-analysis. Crit Care 2015; 19: R 167.

[51] Pradelli L, Mayer K, Muscaritoli M, et al. n-3 fatty acid enriched parenteral nutrition regimens in elective surgical and ICU patients: a meta-analysis. Crit Care 2012; 16: R 184.

[52] Palmer AJ, Ho CKM, Ajibola O, et al. The role of ω-3 fatty acid supplemented parenteral nutrition in critical illness in adults: a systematic review and meta-analysis. Crit Care Med 2013; 41: 307-316.

[53] Singer P, Berger MM, Van den BG, et al. ESPEN guidelines on parenteral nutrition: intensive care. Clin Nutr 2009; 28: 387-400.

[54] Dhaliwal R, Cahill N, Lemieux M, et al. The Canadian critical care nutrition guidelines in 2013: an update on current recommendations and implementation strategies. Nutr Clin Pract 2014; 29: 29-43.

[55] McClave SA, Taylor BE, Martindale RG, et al. Guidelines for the provision and assessment of nutrition support therapy in the adult critically ill patient. Society of Critical Care Medicine (SCCM) and American Society for Parenteral and Enteral Nutrition (ASPEN). JPEN J Parenter Enteral Nutr 2016; 40: 159-211.

[56] Manzanares W, Dhalival R, Jurewitsch B, et al. Alternative lipid emulsions in the critically ill: a systematic review of the evidence. Intensive Care Med 2013; 39(10): 1683-1694.

[57] Cahill NE, Dhaliwal R, Day AG, et al. Nutrition therapy in the critical care setting: what is 'best achievable' practice? An international multicenter observational study. Crit Care Med 2010; 38(2): 395-401.

[58] Tian H, Yao X, Zeng R, et al. Safety and efficacy of a new parenteral lipid emulsion (SMOF) for surgical patients: a systematic review and meta-analysis of randomized controlled trials. Nutr Rev 2013; 71: 815-821.

[59] Heys SD, Walker LG, Smith I, et al. Enteral nutritional supplementation with key nutrients in patients with critical illness and cancer: a meta-analysis of randomized controlled clinical trials. Ann Surg 1999; 229(4): 467-477.

[60] Heyland DK, Novak F, Drover JW, et al. Should immunonutrition become routine in critically ill patients? A systematic review of the evidence. JAMA 2001; 286(8): 944-953.

[61] Tao W, Li P-S, Shen Z, et al. Effects of omega-3 fatty acid nutrition on mortality in septic patients: a meta-analysis of randomized controlled trials. BMC Anesthesiol 2016; 16: 39, doi: 10.1186/s12871-016-0200-7.

[62] Huston JM, Tracey KJ. The pulse of inflammation: heart rate variability, the cholinergic anti-inflammatory pathway and implications for therapy. J Intern Med 2011; 269: 45-53.

Section 5

Kidney Injury in Sepsis

Chapter 5

Sepsis-associated Acute Kidney Injury

Wiwat Chancharoenthana,

Asada Leelahavanichkul and Somchai Eiam-Ong

Additional information is available at the end of the chapter

http://dx.doi.org/10.5772/intechopen.69612

Abstract

Sepsis is a life-threatening condition caused by a dysregulated immune response to infection. Interestingly, sepsis mortality increases with acute kidney injury (AKI) and patients with AKI worsen with sepsis. It is interesting to note that most of the clinical trials on sepsis treatment that derived from the results of translational researches are a failure. This is, in part, because of the complexity of human sepsis in comparison with animal models. Another reason for the failure-translation might be the improper matching of the animal models to the individual patient. It is possible that the main mechanism of sepsis induction in each patient with the variety causes of sepsis might be different. Indeed, immune response to sepsis depends on genetic background, route of immune activation, and organisms. Thus, sepsis treatment classified by "mechanistic approach" to individual patient might be more proper than the classification with "sepsis severity". Specific treatment of sepsis in individual patient according to the specific immune response characteristic might be a more proper translational strategy. Indeed, the understanding in immune response pattern of sepsis and sepsis pathophysiology is necessary for "sepsis mechanistic approach". Then, we conclude most of the topics and our hypothesis regarding SA-AKI in this review.

Keywords: sepsis-acute kidney injury, immune responses, pathophysiology, sepsis mechanistic approach, individual treatment

INTECH
open science | open minds

© 2017 The Author(s). Licensee InTech. This chapter is distributed under the terms of the Creative Commons Attribution License (http://creativecommons.org/licenses/by/3.0), which permits unrestricted use, distribution, and reproduction in any medium, provided the original work is properly cited.

1. Introduction

Sepsis is a condition with life-threatening organ dysfunction caused by a dysregulated host response to systemic infection [1]. Sepsis is the leading cause of acute kidney injury (AKI) in critically ill patients especially in the intensive care unit (ICU). The morbidity and mortality of patients with sepsis-associated AKI (SA-AKI) is still high despite an advance in supportive care [2, 3]. Therefore, a well understanding of SA-AKI is essential not only for nephrologists but also for all physicians to enhance awareness and proper initiation of managements. In this chapter, we discuss several topics in SA-AKI, including the potential new therapeutic managements.

2. Definition and classification

Because SA-AKI definition follows the definition of AKI, in general, the understanding in AKI definition is necessary. Despite the heterogeneity in AKI definition with more than 35 equivalent terms within the last few decades [4], RIFLE (Risk, Injury, Failure, Loss of kidney function, End-stage kidney disease) and AKIN (Acute Kidney Injury Network) classification systems, published in 2004 and 2007, respectively, are widely accepted [5]. RIFLE classification stratifies AKI according to AKI severity as determined by serum creatinine (SCr) or glomerular filtration rate (GFR) and urine output (UO) into three categories; Risk (R), Injury (I), and Failure (F). In addition, RIFLE criteria also categorize advanced AKI into other two categories based on the duration of AKI, kidney function loss (L, persistent AKI > 4 weeks), and end-stage kidney disease (E, AKI > 3 months) [5]. In RIFLE classification, worsening of SCr must be over a 7-day period and persists for at least 24 h. In case of unknown data on previous SCr level, a baseline GFR between 75 and 100 ml/min/1.73 m^2 is assumed, and the modification of diet in renal disease (MDRD) equation is recommended for an estimation of baseline renal function. However, the poor prediction of clinical outcomes from renal function derived by MDRD equation is demonstrated [6]. Therefore, RIFLE and AKIN classifications are modified [7]. In modified AKIN classification, the diagnostic accuracy is improved by precluding either SCr or GFR which discards the requirement of baseline SCr for AKI classification. Despite the improved diagnostic sensitivity of AKIN in comparison with RIFLE classification, AKI outcomes are not in consideration of AKIN system [8]. And AKIN does not synergize with RIFLE criteria in predicting in-hospital mortality of patients with critical illness. Recently, the kidney disease improving global outcomes (KDIGO) work group merges the RIFLE and AKIN classifications in order to establish one AKI classification [9]. KDIGO system defines AKI as an increase in SCr ≥0.3 mg/dL within 48 h or an increase in SCr to ≥1.5 times of baseline SCr or a urine volume of <0.5 mL/kg/h for 6 h. Baseline SCr is the known or presumed value that has occurred within the previous 7 days. In addition, AKI staging of KDIGO follows the AKIN classification with a simplification. KDIGO system shows some advantages over the RIFLE and AKIN classifications in AKI identification and AKI-outcomes prediction. Moreover, KDIGO introduces a new term of "acute kidney disease, AKD" which means the slower increase in SCr or GFR, >7 days but <3 months. This is because renal injury in some conditions progresses slowly and does not match with AKI definition where significant renal function declines within 7 days after the insults.

Regarding SA-AKI classification, Pereira et al. [10] demonstrate that SA-AKI with all of these three classifications—RIFLE, AKIN, and KDIGO—shows similar prediction ability (assessed by the area under the receiver operating characteristic (AUROC) curve) for in-hospital mortality (RIFLE 0.652, $p < 0.001$; AKIN 0.686, $p < 0.001$; KDIGO 0.658, $p < 0.001$). However, the study shows that RIFLE and KDIGO classifications identify AKI more than AKIN criteria. Thus, SA-AKI is AKI induced or enhanced by sepsis which could be classified with any of these three classification systems. It is also interesting to note that SA-AKI is another entity that should be separated from nephrotoxic and ischemic causes of AKI. In fact, inflammatory responses in SA-AKI seem to be more prominent than ischemic and nephrotoxic AKI [11].

3. Epidemiology

A longitudinal, 10 years, cohort with more than 20 ICUs and almost 90,000 patients demonstrates the increased incidence of AKI by 2.8% per year [12]. In parallel, the incidence of sepsis and septic shock is on the rise. In the United States, the retrospective data from 22 years of hospital records reveal 8.7% annual increase in diagnosis of sepsis [13]. Sepsis is the most common contributing factor for AKI. The incidence of SA-AKI is 10–45% based on etiology and population [14, 15]. In surgical condition, the incidence may be as high as 60–70% [16], especially in the ICU setting (>50%) [3]. The severity of SA-AKI also depends on the underlying diseases as well as causes of sepsis [17].

Populations with a high risk of SA-AKI are elderly patients, female gender, and medical comorbidities, including diabetes mellitus, chronic kidney disease (CKD), congestive heart failure, advanced liver disease, and malignancy [18, 19]. In addition, the source of infection and side effect of treatment also contribute as risk factors of SA-AKI. As such, intra-abdominal infection, urological sepsis, infective endocarditis, and blood stream infection are conditions that are susceptible to SA-AKI.

4. Immune responses in sepsis

Sepsis immune responses are very complex and possibly different among diverse etiologies. The progression of sepsis definition is parallel to the current understanding of sepsis pathophysiology in each period (**Figure 1**).

Indeed, the importance of hyperinflammation as a major component of sepsis is gradually altered by the progression in the understanding of sepsis-induced hypoinflammatory responses. The updated definition of sepsis focuses on organ dysfunction, host responses, and infection as an etiology [1]. This is due to the recognition that sepsis in the individual patient is different due to host factors (underlying disease, genetic susceptibility, duration of infection, and organ involvement) and organism factors (virulence and antibiotic susceptibility). Hence, the

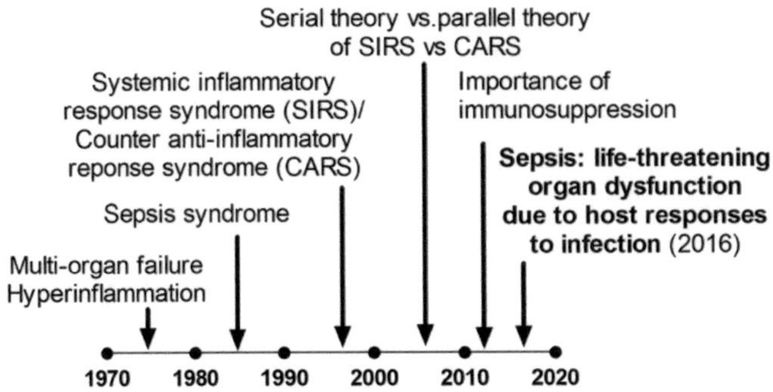

Figure 1. Summary of sepsis definition or main mechanisms in each period.

major mechanisms responsible for sepsis and the proper therapeutic strategies to encounter sepsis for each patient might be different. Indeed, several responsible molecular pathways of sepsis-induced hyperinflammatory response have been demonstrated (e.g., Toll-like receptor 4, Toll-like receptor 9, HMGB1, NF-κB, etc.) mostly in animal models with very rapid clinical progression [20]. These sepsis models enlighten us that the harness of innate immune responses in several processes with adequate organism control attenuates sepsis severity [21–29]. However, the control of innate immune-induced hyperinflammation results in only 50% survival. This demonstrates that other mechanisms might also contribute to the severity of sepsis. Indeed, the clinical observation from patients with sepsis demonstrates immunosuppression in sepsis as determined by (i) high susceptibility to secondary infection, (ii) defect in delayed-type hypersensitivity responses, and (iii) reactivation of dormant virus (e.g., herpes group) [30]. From these clinical observations, immunosuppressive phase of sepsis seems to occur at the late phase. However, Hotchkiss et al. nicely demonstrate the importance of sepsis-induced immune suppression and conclude that moribund stage of patients with sepsis could occur shortly after the onset of sepsis (either hyperimmune or hyporesponsive phase) [30].

As such, the rapid immune exhaustion after sepsis has been demonstrated in mice with the defect of immune inhibition (Fc gamma receptor IIb-deficient mice) [31]. These mice lack the inhibitory signaling with prominent immune responses to infection. The preconditioning with endotoxin induces immune exhaustion and blunt responses of subsequent infection. In translational aspect, this is an example of the rapid immune-suppressive phase that occurs shortly after the onset of sepsis due to the preconditioning in the susceptible host. Moreover, bacterial sepsis also enhances the susceptibility to secondary fungal infection [32]. Interestingly, *Candida albicans* intravenous injection alone and with sepsis causes candidemia after injection at 7 days and 6 h, respectively. Sepsis induces candidemia approximately 1 week faster than non-sepsis control group. This model is also demonstrated that immunosuppression after sepsis could be very rapid, and the host factors are important for the direction of immune responses.

In animal model, sepsis in the pre-conditioning models, pre-existing AKI or CKD or lupus manifestation, demonstrates the more severe hyperimmune responses as shown by the prominent cytokine storms [23, 26, 31, 33]. Then, the host factor is very important for inducing rapid progression due to hyper- or hypoimmune responses in sepsis. While several therapeutic strategies from animal studies are available mostly for controlling hyperimmune responsiveness, the clinical study in sepsis categorizes patients according to the severity of sepsis but not by the characteristic of immune response. Therefore, it is not surprising that nearly all of the clinical studies fail and the difference between animal models versus patients is blamed for the translational failure. The mechanistic-oriented approach with patient characterization by molecular biomarkers, but not simply with sepsis severity, should be more appropriate. Biomarkers for differentiating the direction of sepsis immune response are urgently needed. The anti-inflammatory treatment should be appropriate for patients in hyperimmune response phase and *vice versa* for immunosuppression phage. Moreover, hyper- and hypoimmune response in sepsis is dynamic and the monitoring biomarkers are necessary.

In addition, the molecular-oriented treatment is also an interesting topic in sepsis. For example, anti-HMGB1 should be beneficial in sepsis condition with high HMGB1, and anti-TLR-4 should be appropriate for patients with increased TLR-4 expression on immune cells. Due to the possibility of heterogeneity pathways of sepsis immune responses, the tailor-made or individualized therapy might be the most suitable management of sepsis. However, the understanding in sepsis immune responses is still incomplete. Then, the current sepsis definition depending on sepsis-induced end-organ damage regardless of mechanistic responses is still fragmentary. More studies are needed to reach "sepsis mechanistic approach" in the future.

5. Pathophysiology of SA-AKI

Currently, the pathophysiology of SA-AKI is not completely known. Probably renal biopsy is rarely performed in SA-AKI. Hence, the basic knowledge of SA-AKI is based upon animal models which might be relevant only to a specific condition of SA-AKI in human [34]. For an example, AKI from cecal ligation and puncture model might be relevant to intra-abdominal sepsis but less appropriate representative of pneumonia-induced AKI. The interpretation and results translation from bench to bedside should be properly matched between models and sepsis conditions in patients. Hence, the experiments on the larger animals are performed but, unfortunately, the models might not represent all aspects of patient conditions. With the data gathering from patients and animal studies, the pathophysiology of SA-AKI is, at least in part, through overt inflammatory process-induced renal injury, tubular tight junction (TJ) injury, cell cycle arrest, cellular adaptation/apoptosis, and so on [35]. Perhaps, an alteration in microvascular oxygen transport during sepsis might be the major pathophysiology of SA-AKI. Here, we summarized the mechanisms of SA-AKI mentioned in the literatures (**Figure 2**).

5.1. Microscopic hemodynamic disturbances

The renal microcirculation is an important delivery system of blood and oxygen to kidney tissue. Decreased glomerular perfusion pressure in sepsis is due to microdynamic disturbance with approximately normal renal blood flow (RBF) [36]. However, reduced RBF in sepsis could be found only in some patients with the failure of cardiac output. In fact, sepsis induces hyper-dynamic cardiac responses with relatively high cardiac output. Although RBF is

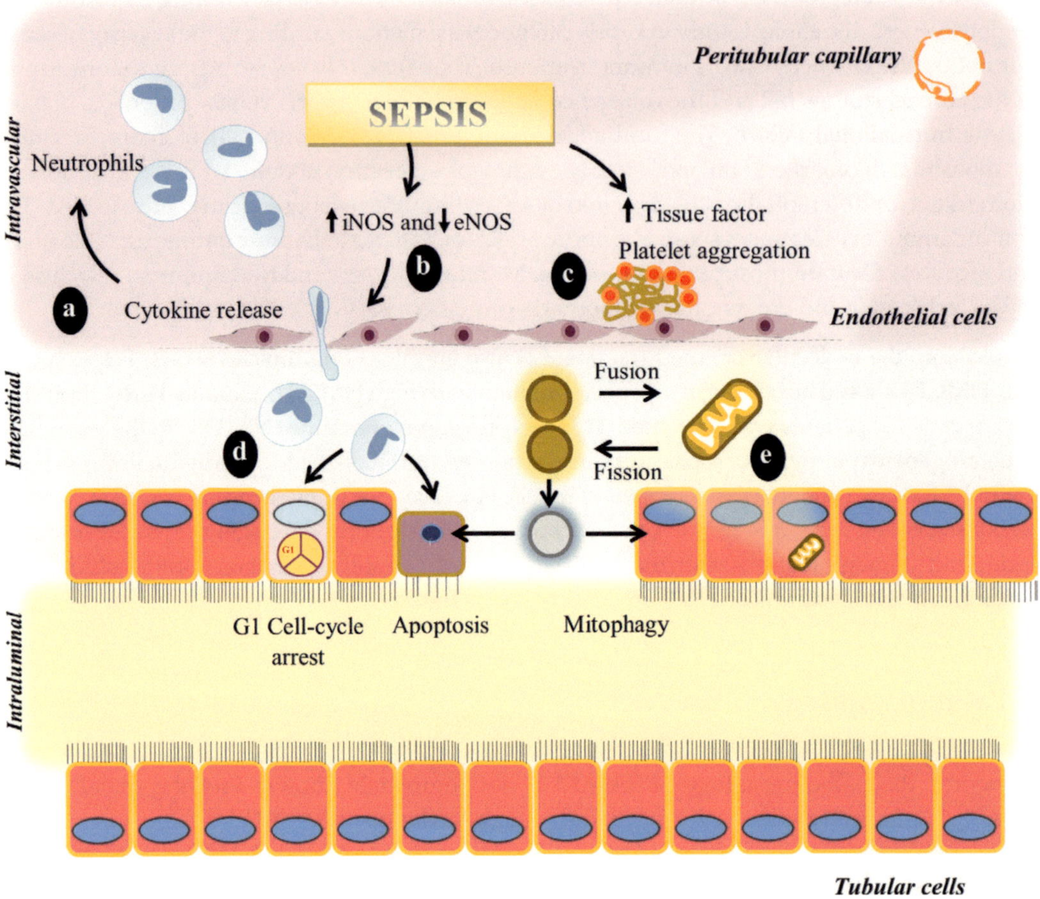

Figure 2. Immune responses in sepsis. Due to renal microcirculation dysfunction (glomerular and tubular capillary), sepsis induces chemotaxis of inflammatory cells and proinflammatory responses leading to endothelial injury (a). Vascular permeability increases due to the downregulation of endothelial nitric oxide synthase (eNOS) activity and induction of inducible nitric oxide synthase (iNOS) (b). In parallel, inflammatory responses increase tissue factor and induce the coagulation system as demonstrated by microvascular thrombosis (c). In addition, inflammatory responses induce tubular cell injury, activate cell cycle arrest at G1 phase and cell apoptosis (d). The insufficient cell energy induces the abnormality in fusion/fission mechanisms of mitochondria resulting in mitochondrial injury (e). The toxic cell environment induced predominant mitochondria fission and dysfunction mitochondria (gray circle). The successful or failure of mitophagy activates cell regeneration or cell apoptosis, respectively (e, lower part).

maintained or increased in sepsis, glomerular capillary hydrostatic pressure is insufficient to permit effective filtration because of efferent-afferent arteriolar imbalance function. Reduced GFR in persistent AKI is a result of several mechanisms including inappropriate activation of tubuloglomerular feedback (TG feedback) [37], tubular back-leak [38], tubular stasis/obstruction, nephrosarca, and altered glomerular permeability.

Normally, TG feedback is controlled by the concentration of chloride delivery to the distal nephron for the induction of afferent arteriole vasoconstriction. Its role is important to limit the hyperfiltration in case of high glomerular perfusion pressure. In SA-AKI, TG feedback is inappropriate due to high chloride presentation at distal nephron because of decreased chloride reabsorption at the proximal renal tubule. This results in overt afferent arteriole vasoconstriction. Marked arteriole vasoconstriction in combination with systemic hypotension causes profound decline in GFR [37].

Tubular cell tight junction disturbance (tubular back-leak) is in the leak-back of non-selective ultrafiltration and ions from renal luminal site into basolateral portion. In SA-AKI, TJ is one of the target actions of endotoxin. Eadon et al. demonstrates direct structural damage of LPS at TJ. The injury of TJ, as determined by the injury at zonula occludens-1 (ZO-1) and claudins, is too severe to explain with LPS-induced-hemodynamic disturbance alone [38]. The tubular back-leak from TJ damage reduces UO by (i) reduced urine volume due to the leaking back of urine into circulation, (ii) increasing intra-renal pressure (renal intracapsular pressure or nephrosarca) [39], and (iii) cell debris-induced tubular lumen obstruction, tubular TJ damage, and abnormal TG feedback mechanisms. The reduction of GFR in SA-AKI also associates with altered glomerular permeability due to inflammation and endotoxins-induced direct glomerular endothelium damage [40, 41]. Nevertheless, the exact mechanisms of glomerular endothelium injury in human remain unknown.

Additionally, an alteration of renal microcirculation might be a physiologic mechanism that aims to limit oxygen and nutrition of organisms. Melican et al. [42] demonstrated, in a urosepsis model, that renal ischemia facilitates bacterial isolation and defends against organisms in sepsis. The suppression of intravascular coagulation by heparin causes fatal urosepsis despite improved microvascular architectures.

5.2. Renal endothelial cells injury

Renal endothelial cells and its function play a central role in microcirculatory dysfunction during sepsis. Sepsis-induced systemic inflammatory cytokines activate endothelium cells and initiate the inflammatory process [41]. Moreover, sepsis induces hypercoagulable state in vessels at both micro- and macroscopic levels. In animal SA-AKI model, Drake et al. demonstrates an increased expression of tissue factor by glomerular endothelial cells in *Escherichia coli* sepsis [43]. The hypercoagulable state in SA-AKI also contributes to localized ischemia and hypoxia in the related intravascular thrombosis area, even though GFR is preserved [42].

Endothelial nitric oxide (NO) synthase (eNOS) induces NO which inhibits platelet aggregation and leukocyte activation. During sepsis, there is depletion of eNOS and activation of inducible NO synthase (iNOS). While eNOS has been shown to attenuate tissue ischemia, iNOS released from activated leukocytes and vascular smooth muscle cells causes vascular dysfunction [44, 45]. Langenberg et al. has recently demonstrated that NOS isoforms increase significantly in SA-AKI, particularly in renal cortex more than in medulla [46]. This may potentially lead to medullary ischemia due to intrarenal shunting.

5.3. Mitochondrial cell dysfunction, autophagy, and apoptosis

Mitochondria are organelles found in every cell and are very prominent in cells of energetic organs including kidney. They are known as the powerhouses of cells. Renal mitochondria are most densely concentrated due to the high and constant demand for adenosine triphosphate. Indeed, lack of cell energy and mitochondrial injury is demonstrated in several organs in sepsis [47]. Normally, mitochondrial dynamics is described as characteristics of "fission"and "fusion."The mitochondrial fission, a cleavage of the defective parts of a mitochondrion, may be important for the maintenance of healthy organelles and necessary for mitochondria distribution to daughter cells during cell division. On the other hand, mitochondrial fusion is the multiple steps fusion between adjacent mitochondria to improve their functions. Both mitochondrial fission and fusion facilitate inter-mitochondria exchanges of metabolites and substrates to maintain the optimal functions that are essential to cell viability [48].

Autophagy is a cellular process by which cytoplasmic organelles are sequestered and delivered to lysosomes for the proper degradation. Therefore, it plays a crucial role in intracellular nutrient turnover, cell differentiation, cellular homeostasis, and viability [49]. But the overactivity of autophagy, however, may cause cell injury or death. In mouse models of SA-AKI, autophagy is rapidly induced and plays important roles in renoprotection [50]. Because mitochondria are prokaryote inhabited inside eukaryotic cell in symbiosis relationship, the breakdown of mitochondria will release several prokaryotic molecules that are capable of inflammatory activation as other pathogen-associated molecular patterns (PAMPs). Hence, the autophagy on mitochondria, as referred to mitophagy, protects unnecessary inflammatory responses and recycles nutrients from the injured mitochondria. In the same line with apoptosis, autophagy is the process that requires enough cell energy. In the condition with the excess injured-mitochondria for autophagy, some mitochondria rupture and mitochondrial cytochrome C further activate cell apoptosis. As such, if there are too many apoptotic bodies to clear by phagocytic cells, apoptotic cells will progress into secondary necrosis where the rupture of its membrane induces prominent inflammation. Hence, mitophagy is also postulated to be another cytoprotective process to control cellular metabolism through the balance in number of mitochondria. Mitophagy is linked to mitochondrial dynamics—fission and fusion—through the surveillance and clearance mechanisms [51].

Taken together, it is conceivable that during the early phase of SA-AKI, mitophagy is increased to control and clear the damaged mitochondria. However, as sepsis progress, the autophagy may be overwhelmed by injured mitochondria, and/or the autophagic processes are disrupted, leads to the abnormal cell functions. Therefore, well homeostasis of intracellular mitochondria to restore healthy mitochondrial mass may be essential for renoprotection and the recovery of renal function in SA-AKI.

5.4. Cell cycle arrest

Cell cycle arrest is a protective mechanism to avoid entering the cell cycle during injury [52], thereby temporarily arresting cell cycle at G_1 stage for reducing cell damage. In cecal ligation and puncture septic model and folic acid-induced AKI, cyclosporine A, a known cell cycle arrest inducer attenuates AKI [53, 54].

In human, Kashani and colleagues propose biomarkers of cell cycle as an early biomarker of AKI [55]; tissue inhibitor of metalloproteinases-2 (TIMP-2), a natural inhibitor of the group of matrix metalloproteinase, and insulin-like growth factor-binding protein 7 (IGFBP7). IGFBP7 regulates the availability of insulin-like growth factor and stimulates cell adhesion. In addition, both TIMP-2 and IGFBP7 are responsible for several molecular pathways, including oxidative stress, detoxification, and inflammatory responses. Therefore, they represent the early stage of any stresses that affect kidney. After tubular cells injury, IGFBP7 directly increases the expression of p21 and p53. Simultaneously, TIMP2 enhances p27 expression through an autocrine and paracrine manners. All of these p-proteins block the functions of the cyclin-dependent protein kinase complexes (CyclD-CDK4 and CyclE-CDK2) during the cell-cycle promotion process. G1 cell-cycle arrest occurs momentarily for avoiding cell division during the injury, and this alarm could send to adjacent cells as paracrine effect. This mechanism needs further exploration. More recently, a new interesting hypothesis mentioned that all of the injuries are the results of the cell maladaptation to an insufficient energy condition [56]. More studies are needed to support this interesting hypothesis.

In the real clinical situations, multiple mechanisms in combination might be responsible for the individual patient. Therefore, a mechanistic approach to patients with SA-AKI needs the integration and understanding of these mechanisms. The biomarkers for detecting these events might be helpful for sepsis mechanistic approach in the future.

6. Clinical approach to SA-AKI

Clinical presentation of SA-AKI is completely uncertain especially in the early phase of sepsis. SA-AKI may develop simultaneously with sepsis or follow by sepsis. Therefore, physicians must be alert of SA-AKI when encountering with sepsis patients and *vice versa*—during evaluation of patients with AKI. In clinical practice, the individual baseline characteristics of patients are very useful for the proper SA-AKI management. Signs and symptoms of sepsis in individual patients depend upon individual susceptibilities and are usually masked by the organ involvement. As mentioned earlier, the SA-AKI diagnosis depends on SCr (absolute increase of SCr concentration of 0.3 mg/dL over 48 h or a relative change in SCr concentration of 1.5- to 1.9-fold to baseline over 7 days) or UO (less than 0.5 mL/kg/h for 6 h). SCr measurement, however, is insensitive indicator of AKI due to the time dependence accumulation. In mice with bilateral nephrectomy, SCr increases from baseline as late as 12–18 h after surgery [33]. According to SCr half-life ($t_{½}$), increments in SCr concentration lag the decrements in GFR by an hour. In addition, sepsis leads to the reduction in muscular production of creatinine from inflammatory process. And diuretic administration in AKI for promoting the non-oliguric phase results in the unreliable UO criteria. Thus, other biomarkers in addition to SCr and UO are required. Urine analysis and urine biochemistry indices may be useful as adjunctive biomarkers to support or differentiate SA-AKI. The presence of urine granular cast and renal epithelial cells is not only for the differentiation between pre-renal AKI and ATN but also for SA-AKI versus non-septic AKI [57]. Urinary sediment examination remains a classic, cost-effectiveness, and worthwhile method for the differentiation of AKI etiologies. By contrast, urine chemistry indices including urine sodium (U_{Na}), fractional excretion of sodium (FE_{Na}), and fractional excretion of urea (FE_{urea}) are beneficial for the differentiation of pre-renal AKI from acute tubular necrosis (ATN) but unfortunately unable to differentiate between SA-AKI versus non-septic AKI. However, Vanmassenhove et al. [58] demonstrates that low FE_{Na} and low FE_{urea} are predictive of transient AKI and oliguria is predictive for impending AKI in early sepsis. Although some studies demonstrate the benefit of urine chemistry indices in SA-AKI, there is still no established urine chemistry test to differentiate SA-AKI from non-septic AKI.

As such, the quest for novel biomarkers as an earlier assessment tool for detecting SA-AKI is crucial. Such biomarkers are categorized into two groups: (i) the determination of renal functions and (ii) the detection of renal cell injury. Some lists of candidate new biomarker of SA-AKI are cystatin C (Cys-C), neutrophil gelatinase-associated lipocalin (NGAL), kidney injury molecule-1 (KIM-1), interleukin-18 (IL-18), liver-type fatty acid-binding (L-FABP), soluble-triggering receptor expressed on myeloid cells-1 (sTREM-1), and activating transcriptional factor 3 (ATF-3). The sensitivity and specificity of these biomarkers vary depending on the timing of measurement and clinical samples. Generally, blood (serum) biomarkers show a lower sensitivity for AKI diagnosis than urinary biomarkers [59, 60]. NGAL is currently the most considered biomarker in AKI. However, it is non-specific to AKI and may be increased by activated neutrophils due to the response of systemic infection. We have demonstrated the benefit of NGAL and Cys-C in SA-AKI with bilateral nephrectomy and bilateral ureter obstruction models [33, 61]. Cys-C is generated from all nucleated cells and NGAL produced from several organs (lung, heart, kidney, and spleen). Because NGAL is reabsorbed from proximal tubules but produced from distal renal tubules [62], NGAL is not only a biomarker of proximal tubular function but also a biomarker of renal injury. Although both molecules are not specific for kidney, NGAL and Cys-C increase more rapidly than SCr after bilateral nephrectomy, possibly due to the more intrinsic sources in the body than SCr. While SCr is generated from muscle due to the utilization of creatine, these molecules are generated from several organs including muscle. It is interesting to note that renal NGAL, as determined by Western blot analysis, after bilateral ureter obstruction, does not increase as rapidly as serum NGAL [33]. This implies the possible limited utilization of kidney-specific NGAL (monomeric form of NGAL) for SA-AKI diagnosis. It is also interesting to note that sepsis does not enhance the production of creatinine, NGAL and Cys-C. SCr and Cys-C after CLP in bilateral nephrectomized mice are lower than CLP in normal mice. And serum NGAL in bilateral nephrectomized mice is not different to the level of CLP in normal mice [33]. In this aspect, among these biomarkers, SCr has several limitations and NGAL is the best representative for SA-AKI in these mouse models.

For other biomarkers, urine IL-18 is a cytokine that respond not only to AKI but also to inflammation and infection. Urine L-FABP has been reported as a good predictor of mortality in patients with sepsis in ICU and shows the significant higher level in SA-AKI in comparison with sepsis-non-AKI [63]. In addition, urine exosome is another interesting source of candidate AKI biomarkers. Exosome is the nanosize vesicle containing molecules from cytoplasm or nuclei surrounded by some parts of cell membrane [62, 64–66]. Exosome is another mechanism of cell-cell communication possibly aiming to deliver non-soluble molecules and/or ligands of cell membrane receptor. As such, MHC-containing exosome could activate other immune cells in a distance without the necessary for the close proximity activation [64]. Moreover, several rapid-degradable molecules (RNA, miRNAs) or molecules of intra-nuclei (e.g., transcriptional factors) could be protected and delivered by exosome. Likewise, our group recently demonstrates the role of urine exosomal ATF-3 as a good additional biomarker for determining the onset of AKI in sepsis [62]. The summary of promising urine and serum biomarkers for SA-SKI is shown in **Table 1**. Although only a single biomarker might be already useful for SA-AKI determination, the combination would be even more beneficial in the clinical practice. For examples, an increase in biomarkers of injury but not biomarkers of renal function could represent subclinical AKI (normal SCr). And an increase in functional biomarkers but not biomarkers of cell injury may represent CKD. More studies are needed.

The discovery of early biomarker of SA-AKI not only improves the clinical management strategies but also adds up the understanding in the pathophysiology of SA-AKI. Unfortunately, SA-AKI pathophysiology in patients is not straightforward. Several comorbidities and the exposure to other AKI inducers (radiologic contrast-media (contrast-induced nephropathy), antibiotics (nephrotoxic ATN or acute interstitial nephritis), and hypotensive state (ischemic ATN) enhance the complexity of sepsis in patients. Hence, the major molecules responsible for SA-AKI in each patient might be different and the different approach and therapies might be necessary. For an example, SA-AKI with the predominant of HMGB1 versus high activated protein C might require the different managements. Therefore, it might be difficult to recognize the molecular responses of SA-AKI only by patient history or current biomarkers. More serum, urine, or tissue biomarkers should be beneficial. Thus, appropriate techniques of renal biopsy in an appropriate time point of SA-AKI might be helpful for an early diagnosis and exploration of the individual molecular responses. This approach could be one of the strategies for "sepsis-individualized therapy." As such, numerous renal biopsy techniques have high yields, safe and effortless [67, 68]. The studies of renal biopsy in the selected case of patients with AKI will be very interesting.

In addition, the interpretation of some non-renal biomarkers in AKI should be cautious. For examples, cardiac troponin I, a biomarker of cardiac muscle injury, is usually high in patients with abnormal renal function [69]. Troponin I of >0.8 ng/dL or the alterations from baseline level or additional use of other biomarkers (e.g., myocardial creatinine kinase; CKMB) might be helpful to determine cardiac cell injury. Fluid status in SA-AKI could affect N-terminal pro-B-type natriuretic peptide (NT-BNP) and troponin T [70]. We also explore microRNA-122 (miR122), a new liver injury biomarker, in several mouse models including sepsis [71]. We found that miR-122 is not superior than alanine transaminase (ALT) for the detection of sepsis-induced liver injury.

Indices	Timing of measurement	AUROC	Threshold values	Sensitivity	Specificity	References (year)
Urine biomarker(s)						
NGAL[a] (ng/mg creatinine)	12-h following septic shock	0.86	>68	0.71	1.0	Martensson et al. [72] (2010)
sTREM-1[a] (pg/mL)	48-h before AKI diagnosis*	0.92	69.04	0.94	0.76	Su et al. [73] (2011)
Cys-C[a] (mg/L)	Within 8 days after admission	0.86	0.106	0.85	0.80	Aydoğdu et al. [60] (2013)
NGAL[a] (ng/mL)		0.80	29.5	0.88	0.73	

Indices	Timing of measurement	AUROC	Threshold values	Sensitivity	Specificity	References (year)
NGAL[a] (ng/mL)	7 days after onset of sepsis	0.86	402	0.89	0.74	Fan et al. [74]
NGAL[a] (ng/mL)	24 h after admission	0.78	350	0.75	0.82	Matsa et al. [75] (2014)
α1m[a] (mg/L)	24 h before AKI onset	0.74	47.9	0.88	0.62	Terzi et al. [76] (2014)
Cys-C[a] (mg/L)	24 h before AKI onset	0.74	N/A	N/A	N/A	Dai et al. [77] (2015)
NGAL[a] (ng/mL)		0.88	N/A	N/A	N/A	
sTREM-1[a] (pg/mL)		0.78	N/A	N/A	N/A	
ATF3[b] (ng/mL)	24 h before AKI onset	0.84	12	0.93	0.85	Panich et al. [62] (2017)
NGAL[b] (ng/mL)		0.64	150	0.98	0.44	
Serum or plasma biomarker(s)						
NGAL (ng/mL)*	12 h following septic shock	0.67	>120	0.83	0.50	Martensson et al. [72] (2010)
Cys-C (mg/L)	Within 8 days of admission	0.82	1.5	0.73	0.68	Aydoğdu et al. [60] (2013)
NGAL (ng/mL)		0.44	N/A	N/A	N/A	
NGAL (ng/mL)	24 h after admission	0.88	400	0.79	0.75	Matsa et al [75](2014)
Presepsin (pg/mL)	Within 24 h of admission	0.70	670	0.70	0.81	Nakamura et al. [78]
Procalcitonin (ng/mL)	Within 24 h of admission	0.88	0.42	0.95	0.65	Nakamura et al. [79] (2015)
Cys-C (mg/L)	24 h before AKI onset	0.74	N/A	N/A	N/A	Dai et al. [77] (2015)
NGAL (ng/mL)		0.83	N/A	N/A	N/A	
sTREM-1 (pg/mL)		0.75	N/A	N/A	N/A	

α1m, alpha-1-microglobulin; AKI, acute kidney injury; ATF3, activating transcriptional factor 3; AUROC, area under the receiver operating characteristic curve; Cys-C, cystatin-C; N/A, data not available; NGAL, neutrophil gelatinase-associated lipocalin; sTREM-1, soluble-triggering receptor expressed on myeloid cells-1.

*No data were available 24 h before AKI onset.

[a]Detection from urinary soluble fraction part.

[b]Detection from urinary exosomal part.

Table 1. Summary of the published studies in early urine and plasma biomarkers for detecting SA-AKI.

7. Managements

Similar to general managements in sepsis, SA-AKI treatment bases upon the rapidly appropriate antibiotic administration and best supportive cares. Here, we summarized the important points in SA-AKI management.

7.1. Fluid therapy

Fluid administration is the corner stone of resuscitation especially in sepsis. Theoretically, fluid responder defines by a patient whose stroke volume (SV) increases by 10–15% after a fluid challenge (250–500 mL) [80], but less than 40% of septic patients are fluid responders [81]. According to Frank-Starling principle, as the preload increases, SV increases until the optimal preload is achieved. Thus, if the fluid challenge does not increase SV, the amount of volume loading would be harmful from the increase in arterial pressure, venous pressure, and, in the end, pulmonary hydrostatic pressures. Moreover, these responses stimulate the release of natriuretic peptide that induces fluid shift from intravascular portion into interstitial space. Of note, kidney is also particularly affected by increased venous pressure resulting in increased renal subcapsular pressure and decreased GFR.

"Fluid expansion as supportive therapy" (FEAST) is the most explicit study that demonstrates the harmful of fluid loading in sepsis [82]. In this randomized study, aggressive fluid loading is associated with an increased risk of death. After the concept of early aggressive fluid resuscitation—"early goal directed therapy" (EGDT)—published in 2001 [83], a number of studies using EGDT protocol have been published subsequently [84–86]. Interestingly, these studies show an obvious reduction in mortality rate, especially during 2010–2015, which associates with the decline in the volume of fluid resuscitation in the first 72 h. Although the fluid resuscitation in an early phase of sepsis with a significant decrease in effective circulatory volume sounds reasonable, the ongoing fluid maintenance therapy remains in trouble, particularly in SA-AKI [87]. Fluid therapy, moreover, is not only incapable of effective reverse septic shock but also contribute to the more renal dysfunction through several mechanisms. For instance, an increased venous pressure following fluid therapy directly increases pressure in renal interstitium and peritubular area in animal models [88]. Because a large fluid bolus (20–30 mL/kg) is associated with volume overload, the approach with the less volume of fluid bolus (200–500 mL) is currently recommended [89]. Acute dialysis quality initiative (ADQI) suggests the approach of fluid therapy in sepsis by dividing into four stages: rescue, optimization, stabilization, and de-escalation [5]. High-volume resuscitation is needed during the rescue stage followed by optimization and stabilization protocol depending on the individual patient. After that, the de-escalation consists of reduced total fluid water in patients where diuretics and/or renal replacement therapy (RRT) might be necessary. Regarding fluid therapy monitoring, passive leg-raising maneuver (PLR) after fluid bolus combined with the real-time SV measurement is the only procedure with a high clinical accuracy of fluid status [80, 89]. Due to the availability of ultrasonography in most of the ICUs, the exclusion of fluid overload by the real-time detection of B-line and abnormal curtain sign in the lung, the vena cava collapsibility by M-mode ultrasonography, and the abnormalities in cardiac function is noninvasive and might be helpful as the additional information in the real clinical situation. But these procedures are operator dependent that need a special training. Nevertheless, physical examination, central venous pressure (CVP), central venous oxygen saturation ($ScvO_2$), chest radiography, and the vena-caval collapsibility index by ultrasonography show limited value in fluid monitoring and is not generally recommended for fluid challenge purpose [90–92]. It might be important to note that in patients with previous normal blood pressure, the mean arterial pressure (MAP) at 65–70 mmHg might be adequate for maintaining renal perfusion. But MAP at 80–85 mmHg might be needed in patient with a history of hypertension [93]. Moreover, serum lactate should be less than 2 mmol/L. The new definition of septic shock from the Third International Consensus Definitions for Sepsis and Septic Shock (Sepsis-3), the stage with the need of vasopressor from maintaining MAP ≥65 mmHg and serum lactate more than 2 mmol/L, implies the importance of serum lactate and vasopressor in clinical practice [1].

In addition to the amount of volume, fluid composition is another issue that must be considered in SA-AKI. Normal saline (0.9% NaCl), a non-physiologic solution, is possibly less beneficial in SA-AKI than other new fluid preparations. Normal saline causes a hyperchloremic metabolic acidosis resulting in decreased renal blood flow (by activation of TG feedback mechanisms and afferent vasoconstriction) and increases the risk of further renal injury [94, 95]. Moreover, normal saline is associated with an increased risk of death in comparison with physiologic salts solution. Similarly, synthetic hydroxyethyl starch is potentially nephrotoxic and not recommended in SA-AKI patients [96]. Blood transfusion is used to improve microcirculatory hemoglobin and tissue oxygenation. However, the results of blood transfusion in reducing morbidity and mortality remain inconclusive [96, 97]. Despite theoretical disadvantage of normal saline in SA-AKI, the result from randomized control trial is still controversy. Moreover, normal saline is generally available in a reasonable price worldwide. Thus, normal saline should still be a main fluid replacement used in SA-AKI. However, the alternative administration of normal saline with other fluid preparations or the limited volume of normal saline might be more beneficial. Recently, Steward approach on acid-base proposed the ratio of serum chloride/sodium (S_{Cl}/S_{Na}) at higher than 0.76 as the indication of chloride access and the timing for the replacement of normal saline into other solutions [98]. More studies are needed.

7.2. Control of acidosis

Acidosis is common in patients with sepsis which might be due to lactic acidosis, respiratory acidosis, and/or hyperchloremic metabolic acidosis from high volume of normal saline. But bicarbonate treatment is not recommended unless blood pH is lower than 7.15. Sodium bicarbonate infusion leads to hypernatremia, hypervolemia, intracellular shift of calcium-induced hypocalcemia, intracellular acidosis, and impaired oxygen delivery [99]. Improved tissue perfusion, proper respiratory machine adjustment, and balance administration of high-volume normal saline with other fluid therapy (e.g., other balance solutions) should be helpful. Tris-hydroxy methyl amino methane (THAM), a weak base with intracellular diffusion, might be beneficial due to the lower intracellular acidosis in comparison with bicarbonate infusion. However, THAM causes hyperkalemia, hypoglycemia, pseudohyponatremia, and increased osmolol gap in patients with preexisting renal dysfunction due to the excretion through kidney [100].

7.3. Antibiotics and other nephrotoxic

The rapid control organism is still the main theme of sepsis treatment. The survival rate of patients with sepsis declines 7.6% for every hour of delayed appropriate antibiotic treatment [101]. Regarding AKI from antibiotic, vancomycin is reported to induce AKI despite appropriate therapeutic level (15–20 mg/dL; the recommended level for the treatment of methicillin-resistance *Staphylococcus aureus* (MRSA)). Vancomycin is also reported to enhance nephrotoxic of piperacillin-tazobactam [102]. Although these events might be due to the contaminants, vancomycin administration in a high dose should be careful and blood level monitoring might be helpful. Other unnecessary nephrotoxic substances, such as amphotericin B, iodinated contrast agents, and so on, should be avoided. In addition, there is only a report of gadolinium (a contrast for MRI)-induced AKI [103] but several reports on increase incidence of nephrogenic systemic fibrosis in gadolinium injection in patients with preexisting renal injury.

7.4. Vasopressors

In SA-AKI, the alteration of vascular tone is a major cause of hypotension and renal injury. Norepinephrine maintains mean arterial pressure and increases renal medullary circulation without RBF alteration leading to improved renal function both in animal models and in human [93, 104–106]. Norepinephrine also restores normal capillary velocity and filtration pressure [107]. Thus, norepinephrine is the first-line drug for septic shock. On the other hand, iloprost, a vasodilatory prostacyclin, has been considered to reduce cortical microcirculatory hypoxia and preserve renal function in animal model of SA-AKI [108]. But the clinical data on the efficacy and safety of iloprost administration are still limited.

7.5. Renal replacement therapy

The general four concerning aspects of renal replacement therapy (indications, timing, modality, and delivered dose) and the traditional clinical indications of RRT ("A-E-I-O-U"; A-acidosis, E-electrolyte disturbance, I-intoxication, O-fluid overload, and U-uremia) should be applied to SA-AKI as other causes of AKI. Indeed, severe metabolic acidosis, fluid overload, and uremia are the top three common indications for RRT in SA-AKI.

Regarding the timing of RRT initiation, the data are heterogeneous, inconclusive, and centers dependence. Although adverse effect of delayed RRT initiation has been reported with a higher mortality rate and worse renal outcome in SA-AKI [109], many consensus guidelines remain set as individual timing based on the only published randomized controlled trial. Bouman et al. [110] demonstrated non-significant differences in renal outcomes or patient survival between early and late initiation of hemofiltration. As such, the recently two large, high-profile randomized trials, specifically designed for the determination of RRT initiation in patients with AKI and critically ill condition, show the discordant conclusions [111, 112]. Single-center early versus late initiation of renal replacement therapy on mortality in critically ill patients with acute kidney injury (ELAIN) demonstrates the benefit of an early strategy of RRT initiation over a delay strategy in the mortality rate of critically ill patients [113]. Although eligible patients are at KDIGO stage 2, they have high sequential organ failure assessment

(SOFA) score at 15.6–16.0. On the contrary, the artificial kidney initiation in kidney injury (AKIKI) study shows a negative result for early strategy of RRT initiation [114]. But patients enrolled in the AKIKI trial are at KDIGO stage 3 with SOFA score at 10.8–10.9 which is lower than the patients in ELAIN study. In addition, SOFA score in the renal component in AKIKI trial is also less than ELAIN study. Therefore, these two studies may have come to different conclusions because of the different inclusion criteria. The patients enrolled in the ELAIN trial are at an earlier AKI stage but more severe sepsis. Nevertheless, another trial for answering the optimal RRT timing is now ongoing—STARRT-AKI (standard vs. accelerated initiation of renal replacement therapy in acute kidney injury) study; *clinicaltrial.gov* NCT02568722.

The choice of hemodialysis (HD) modality for patients with SA-AKI is also important to mention. Although the best choice of HD modality in SA-AKI remains inconclusive, only some studies showed the benefit of continuous renal replacement therapy (CRRT) over intermittent hemodialysis (IHD) in survival and duration before renal recovery [115, 116]. Regarding CRRT in SA-AKI setting, continuous venovenous hemofiltration (CVVH) has recently demonstrated the promising results in comparison with extended daily hemofiltration (EDHF) [115]. Despite more severe sepsis (oliguria and severity of metabolic acidosis) of patients in CVVH group, they have a superior renal outcome on 60-day dialysis independence periods. However, a retrospective cohort study by AlEnezi et al. showed that CVVH does not attenuate mortality and length of hospital stay in comparison with continuous venovenous hemodiafiltration (CVVHDF) [116].

Although the benefit of renal recovery is superior in CRRT, over IHD, owing to the better fluid control with the fewer hypotensive episodes, CRRT is more expensive. On the other hand, on-line hemodiafiltration (Ol-HDF), an intermittent hemodialysis modality that increase mid-to-large molecular clearance by combining diffuse and convective transport with ultrapure dialysate, is a promising alternative modality for SA-AKI. Data from our study demonstrated that Ol-HDF not only benefits in renal support but also offers a potential role in immune modulation in SA-AKI [117]. The comparison of beneficial effects on renal outcomes and patient survival between CVVH and Ol-HDF in SA-AKI patients is ongoing in our center.

In addition, optimal CRRT dose is evaluated in two clinical trials with nonspecific causes of AKI at an effluent rate of 25–30 and 40 mL/kg/h [118–120]. Although there is a tendency toward the reduced mortality rate in the higher dose of CRRT (40 mL/kg/h), it is not enough to reach a significant level. Likewise, the CRRT prescription dose at 30–35 mL/kg/h or 25% addition to the usual dose of CRRT is recommended by some centers to ensure an adequate delivered dose [121]. By theory, delivered CRRT dose over 35 mL/kg/h as known as "high-volume hemofiltration" may remove systemic inflammation and improve septic shock survival, but it is not supported by several clinical studies.

It seems that CVVH has more benefit than IHD only in limited parameters with a significantly higher cost. Hence, we recommend IHD or sustained/slow low-efficiency dialysis (SLED) as a first choice of RRT modality followed by standard dose of CVVH (20–25 mL/kg/h) in SA-AKI depending on patient conditions. In addition, in the area with the limited resources, with less severe sepsis, and/or without other choices of RRT, peritoneal dialysis (PD) might be an alternative RRT modality [122]. However, the adequacy of PD in sepsis and the high glucose level in peritoneal dialysate is the major limitation of PD in sepsis. On the other hand, extracorporeal blood purification (EBP) is currently considered as one of the treatments for balancing homeostasis of sepsis immune responses. The absorption therapy with polymyxin B or other cytokine absorbents shows benefit in hemodynamic parameters and mortality rate in some studies [123] but still inconclusive. Therefore, the specific indication and/or proper biomarkers (i.e., stress-, injury-, functional loss-, and recovery biomarkers) to select patients with the highest probability to be beneficial from any treatment methods are urgently in need [124].

8. Conclusions

Sepsis is often accompanied by acute renal failure, also called sepsis-associated acute kidney injury. The mechanisms by which sepsis and endotoxemia lead to SA-AKI are incompletely understood. However, growing evidences suggest that SA-AKI is a result of sustained renal microvascular hypoperfusion, insufficient cell energy, mitochondria dysfunction, endothelial injury, and cell cycle arrest. SA-AKI is associated with normal or even elevated renal blood flow, which is, at least in part, due to redistribution of blood flow from cortical to medullary region. Fluid therapy and proper antibiotics are crucial managements. Because too much fluid administration in sepsis increase organ dysfunction, hemodynamic-guided approach of fluid therapy and early vasopressor administration in SA-AKI would be beneficial. Currently, the role of renal replacement (RRT) in SA-AKI for renal support and immunomodulation has been evaluated. Although there is no consensus guideline, retrospective clinical studies have suggested that the early initiation of RRT and the use of continuous methods are associated with a better hemodynamic tolerance and renal outcome. Timing and dose of RRT are ongoing debate, yet recently randomized clinical trials remain unable to demonstrate any beneficial impacts of early RRT. In the future, we propose "sepsis mechanistic approach" as an individualized therapy for sepsis and the better matching between the results from the translational researches and the specific patient characteristics.

Author details

Wiwat Chancharoenthana[1]*, Asada Leelahavanichkul[2] and Somchai Eiam-Ong[3]

*Address all correspondence to: aleelahavanit@gmail.com

1 Section of Critical Care Nephrology, Division of Nephrology and Hypertension, Department of Medicine, HRH Princess Chulabhorn College of Medical Science, Chulabhorn Royal Academy of Science (CRAS), Bangkok, Thailand

2 Immunology Unit, Department of Microbiology, Chulalongkorn University, Bangkok, Thailand

3 Division of Nephrology, Department of Medicine, Chulalongkorn University, Bangkok, Thailand

References

[1] Singer M, Deutschman CS, Seymour CW, Shankar-Hari M, Annane D, Bauer M, Bellomo R, Bernard GR, Chiche JD, Coopersmith CM et al. The Third International consensus definitions for sepsis and septic shock (Sepsis-3). Journal of American Medical Association. 2016;**315**(8):801-810

[2] Bagshaw SM, Uchino S, Bellomo R, Morimatsu H, Morgera S, Schetz M, Tan I, Bouman C, Macedo E, Gibney N et al. Septic acute kidney injury in critically ill patients: clinical characteristics and outcomes. Clinical Journal of American Society of Nephrology. 2007;**2**(3):431-439

[3] Uchino S, Kellum JA, Bellomo R, Doig GS, Morimatsu H, Morgera S, Schetz M, Tan I, Bouman C, Macedo E et al. Acute renal failure in critically ill patients: A multinational, multicenter study. Journal of American Medical Association. 2005;**294**(7):813-818

[4] Kellum JA, Levin N, Bouman C, Lameire N. Developing a consensus classification system for acute renal failure. Current Opinion in Critical Care. 2002;**8**(6):509-514

[5] Kellum JA, Mythen MG, Shaw AD. The 12th consensus conference of the acute dialysis quality initiative (ADQI XII). British Journal of Anaesthesia. 2014;**113**(5):729-731

[6] Coca SG, Peixoto AJ, Garg AX, Krumholz HM, Parikh CR. The prognostic importance of a small acute decrement in kidney function in hospitalized patients: A systematic review and meta-analysis. American Journal of Kidney Disease. 2007;**50**(5):712-720

[7] Mehta RL, Kellum JA, Shah SV, Molitoris BA, Ronco C, Warnock DG, Levin A. Acute kidney injury network: Report of an initiative to improve outcomes in acute kidney injury. Critical Care. 2007;**11**(2):R31

[8] Lopes JA, Fernandes P, Jorge S, Goncalves S, Alvarez A, Costa e Silva Z, Franca C, Prata MM. Acute kidney injury in intensive care unit patients: A comparison between the RIFLE and the acute kidney injury network classifications. Critical Care. 2008;**12**(4):R110

[9] Okusa MD, Davenport A. Reading between the (guide)lines--the KDIGO practice guideline on acute kidney injury in the individual patient. Kidney International. 2014; **85**(1):39-48

[10] Gameiro J, Neves JB, Rodrigues N, Bekerman C, Melo MJ, Pereira M, Teixeira C, Mendes I, Jorge S, Rosa R et al. Acute kidney injury, long-term renal function and mortality in patients undergoing major abdominal surgery: A cohort analysis. Clinical Kidney Journal. 2016;**9**(2):192-200

[11] Doi K. Role of kidney injury in sepsis. Journal of Intensive Care. 2016;**4**:17

[12] Bagshaw SM, George C, Bellomo R. Changes in the incidence and outcome for early acute kidney injury in a cohort of Australian intensive care units. Critical Care. 2007;**11**(3):R68

[13] Martin GS, Mannino DM, Eaton S, Moss M. The epidemiology of sepsis in the United States from 1979 through 2000. New England Journal of Medicine. 2003;**348**(16):1546-1554

[14] Hoste EA, Lameire NH, Vanholder RC, Benoit DD, Decruyenaere JM, Colardyn FA. Acute renal failure in patients with sepsis in a surgical ICU: Predictive factors, incidence, comorbidity, and outcome. Journal of American Society of Nephrology. 2003;**14**(4): 1022-1030

[15] Bagshaw SM, George C, Bellomo R. Early acute kidney injury and sepsis: A multicentre evaluation. Critical Care. 2008;**12**(2):R47

[16] White LE, Hassoun HT, Bihorac A, Moore LJ, Sailors RM, McKinley BA, Valdivia A, Moore FA. Acute kidney injury is surprisingly common and a powerful predictor of mortality in surgical sepsis. Journal of Trauma and Acute Care Surgery. 2013;**75**(3):432-438

[17] Rangel-Frausto MS, Pittet D, Costigan M, Hwang T, Davis CS, Wenzel RP. The natural history of the systemic inflammatory response syndrome (SIRS). A prospective study. Journal of American Medical Association. 1995;**273**(2):117-123

[18] Bagshaw SM, Lapinsky S, Dial S, Arabi Y, Dodek P, Wood G, Ellis P, Guzman J, Marshall J, Parrillo JE et al. Acute kidney injury in septic shock: Clinical outcomes and impact of duration of hypotension prior to initiation of antimicrobial therapy. Intensive Care Medicine. 2009;**35**(5):871-881

[19] Oppert M, Engel C, Brunkhorst FM, Bogatsch H, Reinhart K, Frei U, Eckardt KU, Loeffler M, John S. Acute renal failure in patients with severe sepsis and septic shock–A significant independent risk factor for mortality: Results from the German Prevalence Study. Nephrology Dialysis Transplantation. 2008;**23**(3):904-909

[20] Doi K, Leelahavanichkul A, Yuen PS, Star RA. Animal models of sepsis and sepsis-induced kidney injury. Journal of Clinical Investigation. 2009;**119**(10):2868-2878

[21] Leelahavanichkul A, Bocharov AV, Kurlander R, Baranova IN, Vishnyakova TG, Souza AC, Hu X, Doi K, Vaisman B, Amar M et al. Class B scavenger receptor types I and II and CD36 targeting improves sepsis survival and acute outcomes in mice. Journal of Immunology. 2012;**188**(6):2749-2758

[22] Zafrani L, Gerotziafas G, Byrnes C, Hu X, Perez J, Levi C, Placier S, Letavernier E, Leelahavanichkul A, Haymann JP et al. Calpastatin controls polymicrobial sepsis by limiting procoagulant microparticle release. American Journal of Respiratory and Critical Care Medicine. 2012;**185**(7):744-755

[23] Leelahavanichkul A, Huang Y, Hu X, Zhou H, Tsuji T, Chen R, Kopp JB, Schnermann J, Yuen PS, Star RA. Chronic kidney disease worsens sepsis and sepsis-induced acute kidney injury by releasing high mobility group box protein-1. Kidney International. 2011;**80**(11):1198-1211

[24] Nemeth K, Leelahavanichkul A, Yuen PS, Mayer B, Parmelee A, Doi K, Robey PG, Leelahavanichkul K, Koller BH, Brown JM et al. Bone marrow stromal cells attenuate sepsis via prostaglandin E(2)-dependent reprogramming of host macrophages to increase their interleukin-10 production. Nature Medicine. 2009;**15**(1):42-49

[25] Leelahavanichkul A, Yasuda H, Doi K, Hu X, Zhou H, Yuen PS, Star RA. Methyl-2-acetamidoacrylate, an ethyl pyruvate analog, decreases sepsis-induced acute kidney injury in mice. American Journal of Physiology and Renal Physiology 2008;**295**(6):F1825-1835

[26] Doi K, Leelahavanichkul A, Hu X, Sidransky KL, Zhou H, Qin Y, Eisner C, Schnermann J, Yuen PS, Star RA. Pre-existing renal disease promotes sepsis-induced acute kidney injury and worsens outcome. Kidney International. 2008;**74**(8):1017-1025

[27] Doi K, Hu X, Yuen PS, Leelahavanichkul A, Yasuda H, Kim SM, Schnermann J, Jonassen TE, Frokiaer J, Nielsen S et al. AP214, an analogue of alpha-melanocyte-stimulating hormone, ameliorates sepsis-induced acute kidney injury and mortality. Kidney International. 2008;**73**(11):1266-1274

[28] Yasuda H, Leelahavanichkul A, Tsunoda S, Dear JW, Takahashi Y, Ito S, Hu X, Zhou H, Doi K, Childs R et al. Chloroquine and inhibition of Toll-like receptor 9 protect from sepsis-induced acute kidney injury. American Journal of Physiology. Renal Physiology. 2008;**294**(5):F1050–F1058

[29] Dear JW, Leelahavanichkul A, Aponte A, Hu X, Constant SL, Hewitt SM, Yuen PS, Star RA. Liver proteomics for therapeutic drug discovery: Inhibition of the cyclophilin receptor CD147 attenuates sepsis-induced acute renal failure. Critical Care Medicine. 2007;**35**(10):2319-2328

[30] Hotchkiss RS, Monneret G, Payen D. Immunosuppression in sepsis: A novel understanding of the disorder and a new therapeutic approach. The Lancet Infectious Diseases. 2013;**13**(3):260-268

[31] Ondee T, Surawut S, Taratummarat S, Hirankan N, Palaga T, Pisitkun P, Pisitkun T, Leelahavanichkul A. FC gamma receptor IIB deficient mice: A lupus model with increased endotoxin tolerance-related sepsis susceptibility. Shock. 2016

[32] Leelahavanichkul A, Somparn P, Bootprapan T, Tu H, Tangtanatakul P, Nuengjumnong R, Worasilchai N, Tiranathanagul K, Eiam-ong S, Levine M et al. High-dose ascorbate with low-dose amphotericin B attenuates severity of disease in a model of the reappearance of candidemia during sepsis in the mouse. American Journal of Physiology. Regulatory, Integrative and Comparative Physiology. 2015;**309**(3):R223–R234

[33] Leelahavanichkul A, Somparn P, Issara-Amphorn J, Eiam-ong S, Avihingsanon Y, Hirankarn N, Srisawat N. Serum neutrophil gelatinase associated lipocalin (NGAL) outperforms serum creatinine in detecting sepsis-induced acute kidney injury, experiments on bilateral nephrectomy and bilateral ureter obstruction mouse models. Shock. 2016;**45**(5):570-576

[34] Heyman SN, Lieberthal W, Rogiers P, Bonventre JV. Animal models of acute tubular necrosis. Current Opinion in Critical Care. 2002;**8**(6):526-534

[35] Sharfuddin AA, Molitoris BA. Pathophysiology of ischemic acute kidney injury. Nature Review Nephrology. 2011;**7**(4):189-200

[36] Langenberg C, Wan L, Egi M, May CN, Bellomo R. Renal blood flow and function during recovery from experimental septic acute kidney injury. Intensive Care Medicine. 2007;**33**(9):1614-1618

[37] Singh P, Okusa MD. The role of tubuloglomerular feedback in the pathogenesis of acute kidney injury. Contributions to Nephrology. 2011;**174**:12-21

[38] Eadon MT, Hack BK, Xu C, Ko B, Toback FG, Cunningham PN. Endotoxemia alters tight junction gene and protein expression in the kidney. American Journal of Physiology. Renal Physiology. 2012;**303**(6):F821–F830

[39] Herrler T, Tischer A, Meyer A, Feiler S, Guba M, Nowak S, Rentsch M, Bartenstein P, Hacker M, Jauch KW. The intrinsic renal compartment syndrome: New perspectives in kidney transplantation. Transplantation. 2010;**89**(1):40-46

[40] Xu C, Chang A, Hack BK, Eadon MT, Alper SL, Cunningham PN. TNF-mediated damage to glomerular endothelium is an important determinant of acute kidney injury in sepsis. Kidney International. 2014;**85**(1):72-81

[41] De Backer D, Creteur J, Preiser JC, Dubois MJ, Vincent JL. Microvascular blood flow is altered in patients with sepsis. American Journal of Respiratory and Critical Care Medicine. 2002;**166**(1):98-104

[42] Melican K, Boekel J, Mansson LE, Sandoval RM, Tanner GA, Kallskog O, Palm F, Molitoris BA, Richter-Dahlfors A. Bacterial infection-mediated mucosal signalling induces local renal ischaemia as a defence against sepsis. Cell Microbiology. 2008;**10**(10):1987-1998

[43] Drake TA, Cheng J, Chang A, Taylor FB, Jr. Expression of tissue factor, thrombomodulin, and E-selectin in baboons with lethal Escherichia coli sepsis. American Journal of Pathology. 1993;**142**(5):1458-1470

[44] He X, Su F, Velissaris D, Salgado DR, de Souza Barros D, Lorent S, Taccone FS, Vincent JL, De Backer D. Administration of tetrahydrobiopterin improves the microcirculation and outcome in an ovine model of septic shock. Critical Care Medicine. 2012;**40**(10):2833-2840

[45] Legrand M, Almac E, Mik EG, Johannes T, Kandil A, Bezemer R, Payen D, Ince C. L-NIL prevents renal microvascular hypoxia and increase of renal oxygen consumption after ischemia-reperfusion in rats. American Journal of Physiology. Renal Physiology. 2009;**296**(5):F1109–F1117

[46] Langenberg C, Gobe G, Hood S, May CN, Bellomo R. Renal histopathology during experimental septic acute kidney injury and recovery. Critical Care Medicine. 2014; **42**(1):e58-67

[47] Brealey D, Brand M, Hargreaves I, Heales S, Land J, Smolenski R, Davies NA, Cooper CE, Singer M. Association between mitochondrial dysfunction and severity and outcome of septic shock. Lancet. 2002;**360**(9328):219-223

[48] Zhan M, Brooks C, Liu F, Sun L, Dong Z. Mitochondrial dynamics: Regulatory mechanisms and emerging role in renal pathophysiology. Kidney International. 2013;**83**(4): 568-581

[49] Levine B, Kroemer G. Autophagy in the pathogenesis of disease. Cell. 2008;**132**(1):27-42

[50] Howell GM, Gomez H, Collage RD, Loughran P, Zhang X, Escobar DA, Billiar TR, Zuckerbraun BS, Rosengart MR. Augmenting autophagy to treat acute kidney injury during endotoxemia in mice. PLoS One. 2013;**8**(7):e69520

[51] Youle RJ, Narendra DP. Mechanisms of mitophagy. Nature Reviews Molecular Cell Biology. 2011;**12**(1):9-14

[52] Jaeschke H. Mechanisms of Liver Injury. II. Mechanisms of neutrophil-induced liver cell injury during hepatic ischemia-reperfusion and other acute inflammatory conditions. American Journal of Physiolpgy. Gastrointestinal and Liver Physiology. 2006; **290**(6):G1083–G1088

[53] Wen X, Peng Z, Li Y, Wang H, Bishop JV, Chedwick LR, Singbartl K, Kellum JA. One dose of cyclosporine A is protective at initiation of folic acid-induced acute kidney injury in mice. Nephrology Dialysis Transplantation. 2012;**27**(8):3100-3109

[54] Peng ZG, Tian J. Higher serum trough levels of tacrolimus increase 5-year allograft survival in antibody positive renal transplant patients. Clinical Transplantation. 2014: **30**;209-214

[55] Kashani K, Al-Khafaji A, Ardiles T, Artigas A, Bagshaw SM, Bell M, Bihorac A, Birkhahn R, Cely CM, Chawla LS et al. Discovery and validation of cell cycle arrest biomarkers in human acute kidney injury. Critical Care. 2013;**17**(1):R25

[56] Gomez H, Kellum JA, Ronco C. Metabolic reprogramming and tolerance during sepsis-induced AKI. Nature Review Nephrology. 2017

[57] Bagshaw SM, Haase M, Haase-Fielitz A, Bennett M, Devarajan P, Bellomo R. A prospective evaluation of urine microscopy in septic and non-septic acute kidney injury. Nephrology Dialysis Transplantation. 2012;**27**(2):582-588

[58] Vanmassenhove J, Glorieux G, Hoste E, Dhondt A, Vanholder R, Van Biesen W. Urinary output and fractional excretion of sodium and urea as indicators of transient versus intrinsic acute kidney injury during early sepsis. Critical Care. 2013;**17**(5):R234

[59] Di Nardo M, Ficarella A, Ricci Z, Luciano R, Stoppa F, Picardo S, Picca S, Muraca M, Cogo P. Impact of severe sepsis on serum and urinary biomarkers of acute kidney injury in critically ill children: An observational study. Blood Purification. 2013;**35**(1-3):172-176

[60] Aydogdu M, Gursel G, Sancak B, Yeni S, Sari G, Tasyurek S, Turk M, Yuksel S, Senes M, Ozis TN. The use of plasma and urine neutrophil gelatinase associated lipocalin (NGAL) and cystatin C in early diagnosis of septic acute kidney injury in critically ill patients. Disease Markers. 2013;**34**(4):237-246

[61] Leelahavanichkul A, Souza AC, Street JM, Hsu V, Tsuji T, Doi K, Li L, Hu X, Zhou H, Kumar P et al. Comparison of serum creatinine and serum cystatin C as biomarkers to detect sepsis-induced acute kidney injury and to predict mortality in CD-1 mice. American Journal of Physiology. Renal Physiology. 2014;**307**(8):F939–F948

[62] Panich T, Chancharoenthana W, Somparn P, Issara-Amphorn J, Hirankarn N, Leelahavanichkul A. Urinary exosomal activating transcriptional factor 3 as the early diagnostic biomarker for sepsis-induced acute kidney injury. BMC Nephrology. 2017;**18**(1):10

[63] Doi K, Noiri E, Sugaya T. Urinary L-type fatty acid-binding protein as a new renal biomarker in critical care. Current Opinion in Critical Care. 2010;**16**(6):545-549

[64] Huebner AR, Somparn P, Benjachat T, Leelahavanichkul A, Avihingsanon Y, Fenton RA, Pisitkun T. Exosomes in urine biomarker discovery. Advances in Experimental Medicine and Biology. 2015;**845**:43-58

[65] Zhou H, Kajiyama H, Tsuji T, Hu X, Leelahavanichkul A, Vento S, Frank R, Kopp JB, Trachtman H, Star RA et al. Urinary exosomal Wilms' tumor-1 as a potential biomarker for podocyte injury. American Journal of Physiology. Renal Physiology. 2013; **305**(4):F553–F559

[66] Zhou H, Cheruvanky A, Hu X, Matsumoto T, Hiramatsu N, Cho ME, Berger A, Leelahavanichkul A, Doi K, Chawla LS et al. Urinary exosomal transcription factors, a new class of biomarkers for renal disease. Kidney International. 2008;**74**(5):613-621

[67] Babaei Jandaghi A, Lebady M, Zamani AA, Heidarzadeh A, Monfared A, Pourghorban R. A randomised clinical trial to compare coaxial and noncoaxial techniques in percutaneous core needle biopsy of renal parenchyma. Cardiovascular and Interventional Radiology. 2017;**40**(1):106-111

[68] Chancharoenthana W, Kanjanabuch T, Kittikowit W, Srisawat N, Tiranathanagul K, Praditpornsilpa K, Tungsanga K, Eiam-Ong S. The novel middle part approach ultrasound-guided percutaneous native renal biopsy: A better tissue providing technique. Asian Biomedicine. 2014;**8**(2):203-210

[69] Donnino MW, Karriem-Norwood V, Rivers EP, Gupta A, Nguyen HB, Jacobsen G, McCord J, Tomlanovich MC. Prevalence of elevated troponin I in end-stage renal disease patients receiving hemodialysis. Academic Emergency Medicine. 2004;**11**(9):979-981

[70] Sommerer C, Beimler J, Schwenger V, Heckele N, Katus HA, Giannitsis E, Zeier M. Cardiac biomarkers and survival in haemodialysis patients. European Journal of Clinical Investigation. 2007;**37**(5):350-356

[71] Leelahavanichkul A, Somparn P, Panich T, Chancharoenthana W, Wongphom J, Pisitkun T, Hirankarn N, Eiam-Ong S. Serum miRNA-122 in acute liver injury induced by kidney injury and sepsis in CD-1 mouse models. Hepatology Research. 2015;**45**(13):1341-1352

[72] Martensson J, Bell M, Oldner A, Xu S, Venge P, Martling CR. Neutrophil gelatinase-associated lipocalin in adult septic patients with and without acute kidney injury. Intensive Care Medicine. 2010;**36**(8):1333-1340

[73] Su LX, Feng L, Zhang J, Xiao YJ, Jia YH, Yan P, Feng D, Xie LX. Diagnostic value of urine sTREM-1 for sepsis and relevant acute kidney injuries: A prospective study. Critical Care. 2011;**15**(5):R250

[74] Fan H, Zhao Y, Zhu JH, Song FC. Urine neutrophil gelatinase-associated lipocalin in septic patients with and without acute kidney injury. Renal Failure. 2014;**36**(9):1399-1403

[75] Matsa R, Ashley E, Sharma V, Walden AP, Keating L. Plasma and urine neutrophil gelatinase-associated lipocalin in the diagnosis of new onset acute kidney injury in critically ill patients. Critical Care. 2014;**18**(4):R137

[76] Terzi I, Papaioannou V, Papanas N, Dragoumanis C, Petala A, Theodorou V, Gioka T, Vargemezis V, Maltezos E, Pneumatikos I. Alpha1-microglobulin as an early biomarker of sepsis-associated acute kidney injury: A prospective cohort study. Hippokratia. 2014; **18**(3):262e8

[77] Dai X, Zeng Z, Fu C, Zhang S, Cai Y, Chen Z. Diagnostic value of neutrophil gelatinase-associated lipocalin, cystatin C, and soluble triggering receptor expressed on myeloid cells-1 in critically ill patients with sepsis-associated acute kidney injury. Critical Care. 2015;**19**:223

[78] Nakamura Y, Ishikura H, Nishida T, Kawano Y, Yuge R, Ichiki R, Murai A. Usefulness of presepsin in the diagnosis of sepsis in patients with or without acute kidney injury. BMC Anesthesiology. 2014;**14**:88

[79] Nakamura Y, Murai A, Mizunuma M, Ohta D, Kawano Y, Matsumoto N, Nishida T, Ishikura H. Potential use of procalcitonin as biomarker for bacterial sepsis in patients with or without acute kidney injury. Journal of Infection and Chemotherapy. 2015; **21**(4):257-263

[80] Marik PE, Monnet X, Teboul JL. Hemodynamic parameters to guide fluid therapy. Annals of Intensive Care. 2011;**1**(1):1

[81] Mallat J, Meddour M, Durville E, Lemyze M, Pepy F, Temime J, Vangrunderbeeck N, Tronchon L, Thevenin D, Tavernier B. Decrease in pulse pressure and stroke volume variations after mini-fluid challenge accurately predicts fluid responsiveness dagger. British Journal of Anaesthesiology. 2015;**115**(3):449-456

[82] Maitland K, Kiguli S, Opoka RO, Engoru C, Olupot-Olupot P, Akech SO, Nyeko R, Mtove G, Reyburn H, Lang T et al. Mortality after fluid bolus in African children with severe infection. New England Journal of Medicine. 2011;**364**(26):2483-2495

[83] Rivers E, Nguyen B, Havstad S, Ressler J, Muzzin A, Knoblich B, Peterson E, Tomlanovich M. Early goal-directed therapy in the treatment of severe sepsis and septic shock. New England Journal of Medicine. 2001;**345**(19):1368-1377

[84] Yealy DM, Kellum JA, Huang DT, Barnato AE, Weissfeld LA, Pike F, Terndrup T, Wang HE, Hou PC, LoVecchio F et al. A randomized trial of protocol-based care for early septic shock. New England Journal of Medicine. 2014;**370**(18):1683-1693

[85] Peake SL, Delaney A, Bailey M, Bellomo R, Cameron PA, Cooper DJ, Higgins AM, Holdgate A, Howe BD, Webb SA et al. Goal-directed resuscitation for patients with early septic shock. New England Journal of Medicine. 2014;**371**(16):1496-1506

[86] Mouncey PR, Osborn TM, Power GS, Harrison DA, Sadique MZ, Grieve RD, Jahan R, Harvey SE, Bell D, Bion JF et al. Trial of early, goal-directed resuscitation for septic shock. New England Journal of Medicine. 2015;**372**(14):1301-1311

[87] Prowle JR, Kirwan CJ, Bellomo R. Fluid management for the prevention and attenuation of acute kidney injury. Nature Review Nephrology. 2014;**10**(1):37-47

[88] Li X, Liu M, Bedja D, Thoburn C, Gabrielson K, Racusen L, Rabb H. Acute renal venous obstruction is more detrimental to the kidney than arterial occlusion: Implication for murine models of acute kidney injury. American Journal of Physiology. Renal Physiology. 2012;**302**(5):F519–F525

[89] Marik PE. Fluid therapy in 2015 and beyond: The mini-fluid challenge and mini-fluid bolus approach. British Journal of Anaesthesiology. 2015;**115**(3):347-349

[90] Saugel B, Ringmaier S, Holzapfel K, Schuster T, Phillip V, Schmid RM, Huber W. Physical examination, central venous pressure, and chest radiography for the prediction of transpulmonary thermodilution-derived hemodynamic parameters in critically ill patients: a prospective trial. Journal of Critical Care. 2011;**26**(4):402-410

[91] Marik PE, Cavallazzi R. Does the central venous pressure predict fluid responsiveness? An updated meta-analysis and a plea for some common sense. Critical Care Medicine. 2013;**41**(7):1774-1781

[92] Corl K, Napoli AM, Gardiner F. Bedside sonographic measurement of the inferior vena cava caval index is a poor predictor of fluid responsiveness in emergency department patients. Emergency Medicine Australasia. 2012;**24**(5):534-539

[93] Asfar P, Meziani F, Hamel JF, Grelon F, Megarbane B, Anguel N, Mira JP, Dequin PF, Gergaud S, Weiss N et al. High versus low blood-pressure target in patients with septic shock. New England Journal of Medicine. 2014;**370**(17):1583-1593

[94] Chowdhury AH, Cox EF, Francis ST, Lobo DN. A randomized, controlled, double-blind crossover study on the effects of 2-L infusions of 0.9% saline and plasma-lyte(R) 148 on renal blood flow velocity and renal cortical tissue perfusion in healthy volunteers. Annals of Surgery. 2012;**256**(1):18-24

[95] Kellum JA, Bellomo R, Kramer DJ, Pinsky MR. Etiology of metabolic acidosis during saline resuscitation in endotoxemia. Shock. 1998;**9**(5):364-368

[96] Perner A, Haase N, Guttormsen AB, Tenhunen J, Klemenzson G, Aneman A, Madsen KR, Moller MH, Elkjaer JM, Poulsen LM et al. Hydroxyethyl starch 130/0.42 versus Ringer's acetate in severe sepsis. New England Journal of Medicine. 2012;**367**(2):124-134

[97] Sakr Y, Chierego M, Piagnerelli M, Verdant C, Dubois MJ, Koch M, Creteur J, Gullo A, Vincent JL, De Backer D. Microvascular response to red blood cell transfusion in patients with severe sepsis. Critical Care Medicine. 2007;**35**(7):1639-1644

[98] Adrogue HJ, Madias NE. Assessing acid-base status: Physiologic versus physicochemical approach. American Journal of Kidney Disease. 2016;**68**(5):793-802

[99] Kraut JA, Madias NE. Lactic acidosis. New England Journal of Medicine. 2014;**371**(24): 2309-2319

[100] Hoste EA, Colpaert K, Vanholder RC, Lameire NH, De Waele JJ, Blot SI, Colardyn FA. Sodium bicarbonate versus THAM in ICU patients with mild metabolic acidosis. Journal of Nephrology. 2005;**18**(3):303-307

[101] Kumar A, Roberts D, Wood KE, Light B, Parrillo JE, Sharma S, Suppes R, Feinstein D, Zanotti S, Taiberg L et al. Duration of hypotension before initiation of effective antimicrobial therapy is the critical determinant of survival in human septic shock. Critical Care Medicine. 2006;**34**(6):1589-1596

[102] Meaney CJ, Hynicka LM, Tsoukleris MG. Vancomycin-associated nephrotoxicity in adult medicine patients: Incidence, outcomes, and risk factors. Pharmacotherapy. 2014;**34**(7):653-661

[103] Chien CC, Wang HY, Wang JJ, Kan WC, Chien TW, Lin CY, Su SB. Risk of acute kidney injury after exposure to gadolinium-based contrast in patients with renal impairment. Renal Failure. 2011;**33**(8):758-764

[104] Faivre V, Kaskos H, Callebert J, Losser MR, Milliez P, Bonnin P, Payen D, Mebazaa A. Cardiac and renal effects of levosimendan, arginine vasopressin, and norepinephrine in lipopolysaccharide-treated rabbits. Anesthesiology. 2005;**103**(3):514-521

[105] Albert M, Losser MR, Hayon D, Faivre V, Payen D. Systemic and renal macro- and microcirculatory responses to arginine vasopressin in endotoxic rabbits. Critical Care Medicine. 2004;**32**(9):1891-1898

[106] Burban M, Hamel JF, Tabka M, de La Bourdonnaye MR, Duveau A, Mercat A, Cales P, Asfar P, Lerolle N. Renal macro- and microcirculation autoregulatory capacity during early sepsis and norepinephrine infusion in rats. Critical Care. 2013;**17**(4):R139

[107] Albanese J, Leone M, Garnier F, Bourgoin A, Antonini F, Martin C. Renal effects of norepinephrine in septic and nonseptic patients. Chest. 2004;**126**(2):534-539

[108] Johannes T, Ince C, Klingel K, Unertl KE, Mik EG. Iloprost preserves renal oxygenation and restores kidney function in endotoxemia-related acute renal failure in the rat. Critical Care Medicine. 2009;**37**(4):1423-1432

[109] Liu KD, Himmelfarb J, Paganini E, Ikizler TA, Soroko SH, Mehta RL, Chertow GM. Timing of initiation of dialysis in critically ill patients with acute kidney injury. Clinical Journal of the American Society of Nephrology. 2006;**1**(5):915-919

[110] Bouman CS, Oudemans-Van Straaten HM, Tijssen JG, Zandstra DF, Kesecioglu J. Effects of early high-volume continuous venovenous hemofiltration on survival and recovery of renal function in intensive care patients with acute renal failure: A prospective, randomized trial. Critical Care Medicine. 2002;**30**(10):2205-2211

[111] Zarbock A, Kellum JA, Schmidt C, Van Aken H, Wempe C, Pavenstadt H, Boanta A, Gerss J, Meersch M. Effect of early vs delayed initiation of renal replacement therapy

on mortality in critically Ill patients with acute kidney injury: The ELAIN randomized clinical trial. Journal of Amrican Medical Association. 2016;**315**(20):2190-2199

[112] Gaudry S, Hajage D, Schortgen F, Martin-Lefevre L, Pons B, Boulet E, Boyer A, Chevrel G, Lerolle N, Carpentier D et al. Initiation strategies for renal-replacement therapy in the intensive care unit. New England Journal of Medicine. 2016;**375**(2):122-133

[113] Wald R, Shariff SZ, Adhikari NK, Bagshaw SM, Burns KE, Friedrich JO, Garg AX, Harel Z, Kitchlu A, Ray JG. The association between renal replacement therapy modality and long-term outcomes among critically ill adults with acute kidney injury: A retrospective cohort study. Critical Care Medicine. 2014;**42**(4):868-877

[114] Schneider AG, Bellomo R, Bagshaw SM, Glassford NJ, Lo S, Jun M, Cass A, Gallagher M. Choice of renal replacement therapy modality and dialysis dependence after acute kidney injury: A systematic review and meta-analysis. Intensive Care Medicine. 2013;**39**(6):987-997

[115] Sun Z, Ye H, Shen X, Chao H, Wu X, Yang J. Continuous venovenous hemofiltration versus extended daily hemofiltration in patients with septic acute kidney injury: A retrospective cohort study. Critical Care. 2014;**18**(2):R70

[116] AlEnezi F, Alhazzani W, Ma J, Alanazi S, Salib M, Attia M, Thabane L, Fox-Robichaud A. Continuous venovenous hemofiltration versus continuous venovenous hemodiafiltration in critically ill patients: A retrospective cohort study from a Canadian tertiary centre. Canadian Respiratory Journal. 2014;**21**(3):176-180

[117] Chancharoenthana W, Tiranathanagul K, Srisawat N, Susantitaphong P, Leelahavanichkul A, Praditpornsilpa K, Tungsanga K, Eiam-Ong S. Enhanced vascular endothelial growth factor and inflammatory cytokine removal with online hemodiafiltration over high-flux hemodialysis in sepsis-related acute kidney injury patients. Therapeutic Apheresis Dialysis. 2013;**17**(5):557-563

[118] Bellomo R, Cass A, Cole L, Finfer S, Gallagher M, Lo S, McArthur C, McGuinness S, Myburgh J, Norton R et al. Intensity of continuous renal-replacement therapy in critically ill patients. New England Journal of Medicine. 2009;**361**(17):1627-1638

[119] Palevsky PM, Zhang JH, O'Connor TZ, Chertow GM, Crowley ST, Choudhury D, Finkel K, Kellum JA, Paganini E, Schein RM et al. Intensity of renal support in critically ill patients with acute kidney injury. New England Journal of Medicine. 2008;**359**(1):7-20

[120] Kellum JA, Ronco C. Dialysis: Results of RENAL--what is the optimal CRRT target dose? Nature Review Nephrology. 2010;**6**(4):191-192

[121] Vesconi S, Cruz DN, Fumagalli R, Kindgen-Milles D, Monti G, Marinho A, Mariano F, Formica M, Marchesi M, Rene R et al. Delivered dose of renal replacement therapy and mortality in critically ill patients with acute kidney injury. Critical Care. 2009;**13**(2):R57

[122] Phu NH, Hien TT, Mai NT, Chau TT, Chuong LV, Loc PP, Winearls C, Farrar J, White N, Day N. Hemofiltration and peritoneal dialysis in infection-associated acute renal failure in Vietnam. New England Journal of Medicine. 2002;**347**(12):895-902

[123] Cruz DN, Antonelli M, Fumagalli R, Foltran F, Brienza N, Donati A, Malcangi V, Petrini F, Volta G, Bobbio Pallavicini FM et al. Early use of polymyxin B hemoperfusion in abdominal septic shock: The EUPHAS randomized controlled trial. Journal of American Medical Association. 2009;**301**(23):2445-2452

[124] Bellomo R, Kellum JA, Ronco C, Wald R, Martensson J, Maiden M, Bagshaw SM, Glassford NJ, Lankadeva Y, Vaara ST, Schneider A. Acute kidney injury in sepsis. Intensive Care Medicine. 2017, Mar 31. Doi: 10.1007/s00134-017-4755-7. [Epub ahead of print]

Section 6

Development in Clinical Prognosis and Diagnosis of Sepsis

Chapter 6

Clinical Assays in Sepsis: Prognosis, Diagnosis, Outcomes, and the Genetic Basis of Sepsis

Alice Georgia Vassiliou, Stylianos E. Orfanos and Anastasia Kotanidou

Additional information is available at the end of the chapter

http://dx.doi.org/10.5772/67985

Abstract

Sepsis is the most widespread medical disorder of the intensive care unit (ICU) and the most common cause of death in hospitalized patients. Several endothelium-related molecules have been investigated as potential biomarkers for early diagnosis and/or prognosis of sepsis, providing different results depending on study designs. Therefore, it seems that we are still far from the right combination of sepsis markers to be used in clinical practice. It is more probable that a panel of diverse biomarkers will be more efficient in clinical practice. More recently, the potential use of genetic biomarkers for prognostic purposes started emerging for sepsis, in the form of genome-wide association studies. The successful use of modern molecular diagnostics could enable rapid identification of particularly susceptible or less susceptible individuals, leading to tailored therapeutic treatments.

Keywords: sepsis, biomarkers, polymorphisms

1. Introduction

Sepsis, as defined by the third consensus definitions for sepsis and septic shock, is a life-threatening organ dysfunction caused by a dysregulated host response to infection, while septic shock is a subset of sepsis with circulatory and cellular/metabolic dysfunction associated with a higher risk of mortality [1]. However, in the studies used to establish the sepsis-3 guidelines, patient populations were primarily characterized by the previous definitions of sepsis, severe sepsis, and septic shock [2].

INTECH
open science | open minds

© 2017 The Author(s). Licensee InTech. This chapter is distributed under the terms of the Creative Commons Attribution License (http://creativecommons.org/licenses/by/3.0), which permits unrestricted use, distribution, and reproduction in any medium, provided the original work is properly cited.

Sepsis is the most common medical disorder of the intensive care unit (ICU) and the most frequent cause of death in hospitalized patients; it accounts for 1,000,000 cases and 200,000 deaths annually in the United States alone [3]. Unlike other major epidemic illnesses, treatment for sepsis is nonspecific. The new surviving sepsis guidelines [4], that provide an update to the older guidelines [5, 6], presented statements on early management and resuscitation, limited primarily to support organ function and administration of intravenous fluids, antibiotics, and oxygen. Sepsis is a syndrome, not a disease [7] and it occurs in patients with infection [8]. There are no approved drugs that specifically target sepsis. Drotrecogin alfa (activated protein C), the only approved drug specifically indicated for the treatment of severe sepsis, was withdrawn from the market in 2011 [5, 9].

Hence, in the last several years, the search for prognostic and diagnostic markers of sepsis for their use in clinical practice reached its peak. Indeed, the 2001 International Sepsis Definitions Conference [2] introduced C-reactive protein (CRP) and procalcitonin (PCT) as inflammatory markers in the diagnostic criteria for sepsis. However, the new sepsis-3 definitions [1] recognized that sepsis is a syndrome without as yet a validated standard diagnostic test. Sepsis is recognized to involve early activation of both pro- and anti-inflammatory responses [10] along with major modifications in nonimmunologic pathways such as cardiovascular, neuronal, autonomic, hormonal, bioenergetic, metabolic, and coagulation [11], all of which have prognostic significance. The use of biomarkers for the early diagnosis of sepsis may permit early intervention which may reduce the risk of death. Combinations of pro- and anti-inflammatory biomarkers in a multimarker testing kit may help identify patients who develop severe sepsis before organ dysfunction has advanced too far [12]. Biomarker-guided immunotherapy that is administered to patients at the proper immune phase of sepsis may potentially be a major advance in the treatment of sepsis.

In the first part of the chapter, the most commonly studied biomarkers of sepsis are reviewed for their current uses and diagnostic accuracies, including C-reactive protein, procalcitonin, various cytokines and chemokines, endothelial biomarkers, and lactate. The second part of the chapter will focus on the genetic markers of sepsis.

2. Sepsis biomarkers

2.1. Pro-inflammatory biomarkers (acute-phase)

2.1.1. C-reactive protein (CRP)

Proteins, such as C-reactive protein and procalcitonin, are synthesized in response to infection and inflammation. CRP, named after its ability to precipitate the somatic C-polysaccharide of *Streptococcus pneumoniae*, was the first acute-phase protein to be described and comprises a very sensitive systemic marker of inflammation and tissue damage [13]. Currently, CRP is used as a clinical marker to assess the presence of infection and can help discriminate bacterial and viral infections [14]. Various studies have shown CRP to be a valuable marker for the diagnosis of sepsis [15–19] and disease severity [15, 20]. Besides its use in the diagnosis of

http://dx.doi.org/10.5772/67985

sepsis, CRP has also been evaluated as a prognostic marker. More specifically, in ICU patients, elevated concentrations of serum CRP on admission have been associated with increased risk of organ failure and mortality [21, 22]. There have been studies, however, that have not been able to demonstrate that CRP levels are indicative of survival in septic patients [23, 24].

2.1.2. *Procalcitonin (PCT)*

PCT is a protein consisting of 116 amino acids with a molecular weight of 13 kDa and is a precursor of calcitonin produced by C-cells of the thyroid gland, which is intracellularly cleaved by proteolytic enzymes into the active hormone [25]. In 1993 when its elevated level was found in patients with bacterial infection, PCT became an important protein in the detection and differential diagnosis of inflammatory states [26]. The highest levels of PCT are achieved in acute bacterial infections and sepsis. Since then, it has been widely investigated for its prognostic value in sepsis, and has become the most widely used biomarker in the management of infection and sepsis in Europe [27]. The efficacy of serial PCT concentrations has been evaluated as a prognostic biomarker of outcome in sepsis [28, 29]. PCT clearance has also been extensively studied as a biomarker for monitoring sepsis outcomes; at this end various reports have demonstrated significant improvement in PCT clearance in survivors compared to nonsurvivors in both severe sepsis and septic shock patients [28, 30–32]. A large meta-analysis comprising 23 studies with 3944 patients concluded that PCT nonclearance was a prognostic factor of death in patients with sepsis [33]. Hence, it has been suggested that PCT clearance could be indicative of patient outcome and serial PCT concentration measurements throughout hospitalization could facilitate treatment planning to improve patient outcome.

Several meta-analyses have investigated the value of PCT as a diagnostic marker of sepsis. However, this vast number of studies and meta-analyses has produced conflicting results. Uzzan *et al.* found that PCT represents a good biological diagnostic marker for sepsis, severe sepsis, or septic shock and suggested that procalcitonin should be included in diagnostic guidelines for sepsis and in clinical practice in intensive care units [34]. The findings of Tang *et al.* on the other hand do not support the widespread use of the procalcitonin test in critical care settings [35]. Another large meta-analysis consisting of 3244 patients suggested that PCT is a helpful biomarker for early diagnosis of sepsis in critically ill patients [36]. As far as prognosis is concerned, a meta-analysis of 2353 patients proved that there is a significant difference between PCT levels as early as day 1 between survivors and nonsurvivors among septic patients [37].

The efficacy of procalcitonin-guided antibiotic treatment has also been studied. A meta-analysis of 1075 patients concluded that procalcitonin is a helpful method to guide antibiotic therapy and surgical interventions without, however, exhibiting a beneficial effect on mortality [38]. The major benefit was shorter antibiotic treatment duration.

In conclusion, PCT in some studies has been found to be a superior marker of infection than CRP in critically ill patients, and nonetheless is a useful marker of the severity of infection [15, 39–43].

2.2. Cytokine/chemokine biomarkers

Cytokines are immuno-regulators produced in response to an infection or injury. A more clear understanding of the pathophysiological basis of sepsis, including the pro- and anti-inflammatory response during the hyperinflammatory and immunosuppressive phase of the disease, respectively, can lead to an alternative treatment approach. In septic patients, secretion of pro-inflammatory cytokines at the systemic inflammatory response syndrome or SIRS and anti-inflammatory cytokines, at the compensatory anti-inflammatory response syndrome (CARS) [44], occurs in a simultaneous manner from the very first instant of infection [45]. Mean serum levels of cytokines are higher in septic compared to nonseptic patients. Cytokines have therefore been proposed to be sepsis biomarkers in cases of neonatal and adult sepsis [46, 47]. Interleukin-6 (IL-6), IL-8, and IL-10 are the most extensively studied cytokines in diagnosing sepsis, evaluating the intensity of the inflammatory response and determining the prognosis for the patient. IL-6 comprises a pro-inflammatory cytokine, IL-8 is a major chemokine, and IL-10 represents an anti-inflammatory cytokine.

2.2.1. Pro-inflammatory cytokines and chemokines

Tumor necrosis factor-alpha (TNF-α), IL-1β, and IL-6 are the cytokines that mediate the initial response of the innate immune system to injury or infection. Neutrophils are the first and most important cellular host defense against invading pathogens. Neutrophils migrate rapidly from the blood to the site of infection and this recruitment is mediated by pro-inflammatory mediators, such as TNF-α, IL-1β, and neutrophil-active chemoattractants, like IL-8. Therefore, these cytokines are essentially responsible for the features of SIRS and could be potentially useful as biomarkers of sepsis. IL-6 enhances the liver's production of the so-called acute phase reactants, including CRP, and also stimulates a shift in the production of cells in the bone marrow so that more polymorphonuclear cells (PMNs) are produced. However, it is also possible that the cells entering circulation could disseminate inflammation into other organs, eventually leading to damage [48]. Impairment of neutrophil migration has been described in sepsis, suggesting that in human sepsis, failure of neutrophil migration is associated with a poor prognosis. In human sepsis, lipopolysaccharide (LPS) is known to induce TNF-α production by activating various kinases, leading to NF κB (nuclear factor kappa light chain enhancer of activated B cells) activation.

Levels of circulating cytokines are frequently increased in sepsis [49–57]. IL-6 levels are increased in patients with infectious complications and have been used to differentiate SIRS from sepsis [58]. Studies have shown that high concentrations of TNF-α and IL-6 are predictive of organ failure and increased mortality in septic patients [55, 57, 59]. IL-8 has been used to predict the severity of sepsis in pediatric patients, although the use of IL-8 has not been confirmed in adults [60, 61]. A very recent study showed that the interleukin-1 receptor 2 (IL1R2) might be a better biomarker not only for sepsis diagnosis but also for differentiation of sepsis infected with G-positive or G-negative bacteria compared to PCT, Acute Physiology and Chronic Health Evaluation II (APACHE II), and CRP [62].

http://dx.doi.org/10.5772/67985

In line with this, clinical trials with an anti-TNF-α monoclonal antibody in septic patients did not show any advantage [63]. Interestingly, it was demonstrated in subsequent studies that blocking IL-6 caused a complete inhibition of endotoxin-induced activation of coagulation [64]. Administration of an IL-1 receptor antagonist partly blocked the pro-coagulant response in experimental sepsis models and inhibited thrombin generation in patients [65]. Overall, anti-TNF-α and IL-1β clinical trials undertaken in patients with sepsis have been unsuccessful [66].

2.2.2. *IL-27*

IL-27, a bioactive member of the IL-12 cytokine family, may serve as a useful biomarker in estimating risk of bacterial infection among critically ill pediatric and adult patients [67–70]. Moreover, when used in combination with PCT, IL-27 may improve classification of critically ill adults with sepsis [68, 71].

2.2.3. *Anti-inflammatory cytokines*

Just as described above how the pro-inflammatory syndrome is characterized by many different and sometimes redundant cytokines, the CARS response also seems to involve many cytokines. The most important, however, is IL-10 [72]. It now has been established that IL-10 has multiple immunosuppressive roles [73] with its most important being the downregulation of TNF-α. Poor patient outcome has been associated with increased blood levels of the anti-inflammatory cytokine IL-10 [74]. IL-10 has been shown to protect endotoxemic mice [75–77], whereas in models of polymicrobial sepsis it seems to be deleterious [78, 79]. These inconsistent results likely depend on the time of administration and the severity of infection. Indeed, in view of these contradicting results, studies have documented that administration of anti-IL-10 monoclonal antibodies beyond the initial pro-inflammatory state of polymicrobial sepsis improves survival of animals subjected to sepsis [80], and furthermore, it is the timing and scale of the anti-inflammatory response that predicts severity of infection in murine model of sepsis [81].

To summarize, pro- and anti-inflammatory cytokines and chemokines have some value in the evaluation of the inflammatory response; however, they lack discriminative power to differentiate between infectious and noninfectious systemic inflammation. Elevated levels of pro- and anti-inflammatory cytokines are found mostly in nonsurvivors, whereas reduced levels are found in survivors of sepsis [82]. Even though they play an important part in the pathogenesis of sepsis, the role of cytokines as sepsis biomarkers remains to be established.

2.3. Endothelial proteins as potential biomarkers

Since early widespread endothelial dysfunction and/or damage appear to be directly involved in sepsis [83], there is a strong biological rationale for targeting markers of endothelial activation and dysfunction as biomarkers of the septic syndrome.

2.3.1. *Angiopoietins*

Angiopoietin-1 (Ang-1) and angiopoietin-2 are antagonistic factors that trigger endothelial cell (EC) activation; the role of angiopoietin-1 is to maintain vessel integrity and block vascular leakage, while angiopoietin-2 (Ang-2) counteracts the protective effects of Ang-1-Tie2 signaling [84, 85]. Ang-2 has been proposed as a biomarker in sepsis, since its release directly reflects vascular barrier breakdown [86–88]. More specifically, Ang-2 levels have been found to be elevated in patients with severe sepsis compared to patients with sepsis or not [89–91], higher Ang-2 levels have been reported in septic patients with worse clinical outcome [92–94], and increased Ang-2 levels have been demonstrated in nonsurvivors compared to survivors [95, 96]. Fewer studies have examined the role of Ang-1 in sepsis; those reports have shown either decreased levels of Ang-1 in critically ill patients compared to healthy controls, or have associated decreased levels at ICU admission with higher mortality [94, 97].

2.3.2. *Selectins*

Prior to the firm adhesion of leukocytes to the vascular endothelium and their transmigration to the sites of injury and inflammation, capture and rolling of leukocytes along the endothelium occurs. This is mediated by a family of cell adhesion molecules (or CAMs), called the selectin family [98]. Levels of soluble (s)E-selectin are very low in healthy individuals, whereas increased concentrations have been reported in various inflammatory pathologies [99–102]; other investigations have shown higher levels in nonsurvivors than survivors [103, 104]. Recently, it was demonstrated that sE-selectin levels may be used as predictor of fatal outcome in patients with SIRS [105]. Moreover, sE-selectin has also been proposed as a predictor of bacteremia in severe sepsis patients [106]. P-selectin has a similar function, but is constitutively expressed in lung ECs, and correlates with lung endothelial injury [107]. A recent study by Wang *et al.* [108] demonstrated in patients hospitalized for infections that higher baseline levels of interleukin-6, sE-selectin, and soluble intercellular adhesion molecule-1 (sICAM-1) may differentiate those patients who will develop a mild response to infection from those who will develop full-blown sepsis. A most recent study showed that high levels of the circulating endothelial adhesion molecules sE- and sP-selectin, measured at ICU admission, appear to be associated with sepsis development in time [109].

2.3.3. *Soluble intercellular adhesion molecule-1 (sICAM-1)*

Both the innate and adaptive immune responses depend on the migration of leukocytes across endothelial cells [110]. Specific adhesion glycoproteins are required for the binding of leukocytes to ECs. One such glycoprotein, intercellular adhesion molecule-1 (ICAM-1), controls the firm adhesion of neutrophils on endothelium and consequently their transmigration to the sites of infection. ICAM-1 has been studied as a biomarker of sepsis severity and outcome. These studies have produced inconsistent and conflicting results, possibly reflecting the time

http://dx.doi.org/10.5772/67985

point at which they were measured [105]. ICAM-1 production has been shown to be induced by endotoxins and has been associated with sepsis severity [102, 111] or mortality [111, 112], while sICAM-1 seems to be a reliable biomarker for distinguishing patients with sepsis from those with noninfectious SIRS [105].

2.3.4. Soluble platelet/endothelial cell adhesion molecule-1 (sPECAM-1)

Platelet/endothelial cell adhesion molecule-1 (PECAM-1, CD31) is a 130-kDa cell adhesion molecule that is expressed on the surfaces of leukocytes, such as monocytes, neutrophils, and some T-cell subsets, as well as on platelets and the intercellular junctions of endothelial cells [113]. Serum levels of sPECAM-1 have been demonstrated to be higher in septic patients compared with nonseptic patients at admission and are also higher compared to healthy controls [114, 115].

2.3.5. Endocan

Endocan is a proteoglycan expressed and secreted by the vascular endothelium in the lung and kidney, in response to pro-inflammatory cytokines and pro-angiogenic factors, which inhibits leukocyte migration [116]. The molecule is cleaved through the activity by cathepsin G generating a novel endocan peptide fragment of 14 kDa, named p14, which exhibits higher concentrations in septic patients compared to healthy volunteers [117]. Several studies have shown that this glycoprotein can be used as a strong and significant predictor of sepsis severity and outcome [118–122].

2.4. Receptor biomarkers

2.4.1. Soluble urokinase-type plasminogen activator receptor (suPAR)

The soluble urokinase-type plasminogen activator receptor (suPAR) was first identified in 1985 as a cellular binding site for urokinase [123]. Since then suPAR has been investigated as a potential prognostic marker in the ICU. In critically ill patients, several studies have reported elevated suPAR in SIRS, bacteremia, sepsis, and septic shock, in which high circulating suPAR levels indicated a poor prognosis, including organ dysfunction and mortality [124–127].

Systematic reviews have concluded, however, that the diagnostic value of suPAR in sepsis is limited [128] and suPAR does not appear to be better in diagnosing sepsis compared to other biomarkers, like CRP and PCT [129, 130]. Plasma suPAR levels are, however, a sensitive and specific independent prognostic biomarker in patients with bacteremia. This plasma protein may be used to identify patients who are severely ill with pneumococcal bacteremia, and predict mortality [131–133].

2.4.2. *Soluble triggering receptor expressed on myeloid cells-1 (sTREM-1)*

Triggering receptor expressed on myeloid cells-1 (TREM-1) is an immunoglobulin whose signaling induces the production of cytokines, chemokines, and reactive oxygen species, all of which contribute to the inflammatory response. Furthermore, TREM-1 signaling leads to degranulation of neutrophils and increased phagocytosis. A soluble form of TREM-1 (sTREM-1) can be measured in body fluids and has potential as a diagnostic and prognostic biomarker of sepsis [134–139]. Other studies, however, have not been able to demonstrate sTREM-1 as a single marker sufficient for sepsis diagnosis and prognosis [140–142].

Systematic reviews of the literature have shown that elevated sTREM-1 concentrations have a moderate diagnostic performance in differentiating sepsis from SIRS and were not sufficient for sepsis diagnosis in systemic inflammatory patients [140]. Furthermore, it exhibits a moderate prognostic significance in assessing the mortality of infection in adult patients and sTREM-1 alone is insufficient to predict mortality as a biomarker [142]. However, sTREM-1 represents a reliable biological marker of bacterial infection [143].

2.4.3. *Soluble endothelial protein C receptor (sEPCR)*

The protein C (PC) anticoagulant system provides important control of both blood coagulation and inflammatory pathways [144]. This system also involves protein S (PS), and the endothelial receptors thrombomodulin (TM) and endothelial protein C receptor (EPCR). Conversion of PC to activated PC (APC) is generated by TM-bound thrombin and is drastically augmented by the presence of EPCR [145]. The presence of a soluble form of EPCR (sEPCR) that exists under normal conditions and which is elevated in conditions marked by enhanced inflammation [146], supports the notion of EPCR shedding. While the role of membrane EPCR is clearly antithrombotic and anti-inflammatory, the physiological significance of circulating sEPCR *in vivo* is as yet not fully understood and it is still unknown whether soluble EPCR levels may have a predictive value in the appearance of sepsis.

In previous studies, sEPCR levels in septic patients were found to be significantly higher [146, 147], unchanged [148], or even lower [149] than in healthy volunteers. A study by Kager *et al.* [150] showed that increased plasma sEPCR levels correlate with accelerated mortality in patients with melioidosis, while overexpression of EPCR in transgenic animals aggravates outcome during Gram-negative pneumonia-derived sepsis. In another recent report, early kinetics of sEPCR levels in severe sepsis was correlated with outcome [151], by a proposed mechanism of counteracting the anticoagulant action of membrane EPCR. The authors suggested that sEPCR could provide an early biological marker of outcome in severe sepsis. Vassiliou *et al.* [152] showed that levels of soluble EPCR at ICU admission are higher in originally nonseptic patients who subsequently become septic compared to those who will not.

2.4.4. *Presepsin*

Cluster of differentiation 14 (CD14) is a glycoprotein expressed on monocytes and macrophages, which serves as a receptor for lipopolysaccharides. As a pattern recognition molecule it plays a role in the innate immune system by activating a pro-inflammatory signaling cascade upon contact with microorganisms [153]. During inflammation, protease activity releases soluble CD14 (sCD14) fragments, one of which has been identified as presepsin (sCD14-ST).

Presepsin was discovered as a new marker in Japan in 2002 [154], as a molecule whose levels were elevated specifically in the blood of patients with sepsis, and in the last few years has been extensively studied as a diagnostic and prognostic sepsis biomarker. In 2012, a multicenter prospective study investigated the clinical usefulness of presepsin for discriminating between bacterial and nonbacterial infections and compared it with PCT and IL-6 [155]. The study concluded that presepsin is useful for the diagnosis of sepsis and that it was superior to conventional markers and blood cultures. Ulla *et al.* [153] evaluated the diagnostic and prognostic value of presepsin in the emergency department and found that presepsin was useful in the early diagnosis of infection in a population of patients with SIRS, sepsis, severe sepsis, and septic shock. Moreover, presepsin exhibited a prognostic value, since its initial levels were correlated with mortality. In ICU patients, presepsin demonstrated diagnostic capacity in differentiating sepsis severity and prognostic value in mortality [156], while Masson *et al.* [157] found that presepsin measured on the first day in ICU in patients with severe sepsis or septic shock was higher in nonsurvivors compared to survivors, thus exhibiting useful prognostic importance. In 2015, three large meta-analyses concluded that presepsin has moderate diagnostic capacity for the detection of sepsis and it is an effective adjunct biomarker, but is insufficient to detect or rule out sepsis when used alone [158–160].

Since then, more studies have been performed, comparing presepsin to markers such as PCT and CRP. Results from these studies have shown that presepsin could differentiate between septic and nonseptic patients with comparable accuracy to CRP and PCT [161, 162], while presepsin and CRP showed similar performance for predicting 28-day mortality [161]. In patients with suspected sepsis, presepsin and PCT showed a good diagnostic accuracy in predicting bacteremia and bacterial DNAemia, superior to CRP [163]. In two very recent studies, presepsin seemed to be as valuable a biomarker as PCT or CRP in the evaluation of infectious complications in patients after heart transplantation [164], while another study concluded that the introduction of presepsin in clinical practice is not justified, since although it is a valuable biomarker for diagnosis of infection and sepsis, its diagnostic accuracy does not improve that of PCT [165].

Presepsin has been shown to be beneficial as a sepsis marker in adults. Nevertheless, very few data are available in neonates. Recent studies have shown that presepsin is significantly higher in preterm infants with early onset sepsis (EOS) compared with uninfected infants [166] and that it may be used as a reliable and accurate marker for both diagnosis and follow-up of EOS [167]. Pugni *et al.* [168] provided reference ranges for presepsin as an effective sepsis marker in neonates.

2.5. Lactate

Lactate is currently the most commonly used biomarker to identify sepsis. In the last years, several studies have emphasized the prognostic value of initial lactate levels or lactate clearance [169, 170]. Lactate, apart from being the end product of anaerobic glycolysis reflecting tissue oxygen delivery-utilization, is also increased during stress and critical illness [171]. Elevated serum lactate levels are associated with poor outcomes in diverse populations of critically ill patients, such as multiple organ failure, morbidity, and mortality [172–175]. Clinically, serum lactate is a potentially useful biomarker to risk-stratify patients with severe sepsis presenting to the emergency department [170, 174, 175], so it has been hypothesized that early detection of elevated lactate levels may result in early identification of patients at risk of adverse outcomes [176]. In sepsis these elevated levels may be due to either impaired lactate clearance or excessive production [177, 178]. Two very recent studies [176, 179] utilized serum lactate levels at admission in order to diagnose sepsis in undifferentiated patients with suspected sepsis, emphasizing on the utility of early lactate measurement in such context, while Vassiliou *et al.* demonstrated that combining sE- and sP-selectin with serum lactate offers better prognostic value for sepsis development in initially nonseptic ICU patients [180].

Lactate kinetics has proved a valuable marker for response to resuscitative handlings in septic patients, associated with clinical outcome and mortality. Thus, according to the new sepsis-3 guidelines "patients with septic shock can be clinically identified by a vasopressor requirement to maintain a mean arterial pressure of 65 mmHg or greater and serum lactate level greater than 2 mmol/L (>18 mg/dL) in the absence of hypovolemia. This combination is associated with hospital mortality rates greater than 40%" [1].

2.6. Biomarker panels

Since as yet no single accepted biomarker or combination of biomarkers can be clinically used to diagnose patients with suspected sepsis, the multi-marker or panel approach has been suggested to improve clinical utility. Many groups have studied such biomarker panels. Kofoed *et al.* [181] showed that combining data from several markers improves diagnostic accuracy in detecting bacterial versus nonbacterial causes of inflammation. Another study identified a panel of three different biomarkers that could assess risk of organ dysfunction, shock, and death in emergency department patients with suspected sepsis [182].

Another panel including both pro-inflammatory and anti-inflammatory markers, comprising IL-6, IL-8, and the anti-inflammatory cytokine IL-10 was associated with a worse outcome for patients with sepsis [183]. As mentioned earlier, high concentrations of TNF-α and IL-6 are predictive of organ failure and increased mortality [55, 57], but poor patient outcome is also associated with increased levels of the anti-inflammatory cytokine IL-10 [74]. This apparent paradox is explained by the proposal that infection induces an initial stage of systemic inflammation (SIRS), with elevated blood levels of pro-inflammatory cytokines (e.g., TNF-α and IL-1β), that is followed by a compensatory anti-inflammatory response (CARS) defined by high circulating levels of anti-inflammatory cytokines (e.g., IL-10 and IL-13), and it is indeed the sustained overproduction of the anti-inflammatory cytokine IL-10 that is the main predictor of severity and fatal outcome [184].

Figure 1 summarizes all major biomarkers involved in the inflammatory response in sepsis.

http://dx.doi.org/10.5772/67985

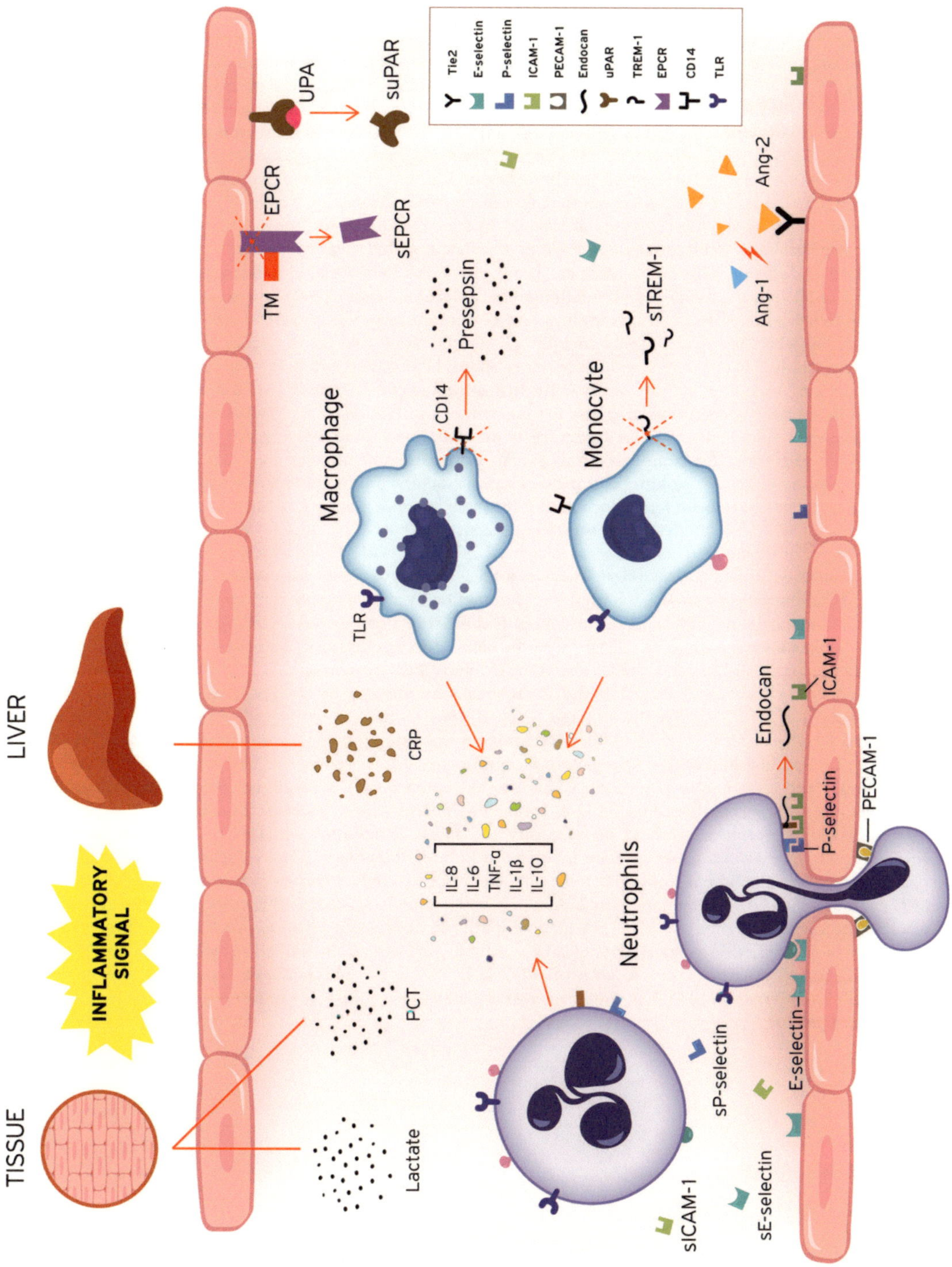

Figure 1. Major biomarkers in sepsis. During the inflammatory response a large number of cytokines, chemokines, and soluble molecules are secreted, affecting coagulation, endothelial activation and dysfunction, and vascular barrier permeability. The result is immune dysregulation and persistent immune suppression. The host immune response to sepsis includes activation of both pro- and anti-inflammatory stages and excessive activation of immune cells. Proteins, such as CRP and PCT are synthesized in the acute phase in response to infection and inflammation. The cells of the innate immune system release large amounts of pro- and anti-inflammatory cytokines, such as IL-1β, IL-6, IL-8, TNF-α, and IL-10, during the hyper-inflammatory and immunosuppressive phase of the disease, respectively, from the very first instant of infection. The high levels of circulating cytokines can potentiate organ damage by endothelial injury and other routes. Ang-2 disrupts the protective effects of Ang-1-Tie2 signaling that maintains vessel integrity and inhibits vascular leakage. In critically ill patients, the release of Ang-2 directly reflects vascular barrier breakdown. Endothelial damage is associated with activation of neutrophils and expression of neutrophil and endothelial adhesion molecules. These molecules help localize leukocytes to the area of injury; however, before leaving the blood vessel, inflammatory molecules released by activated neutrophils can produce additional endothelial injury. Both the innate and adaptive immune responses depend on the migration of leukocytes across endothelial cells. The selectin family, including E-selectin and P-selectin, is an early mediator of the adhesion of activated neutrophils to endothelia in inflammatory states, before their firm adhesion and diapedesis at sites of tissue injury and inflammation. ICAM-1 controls the firm adhesion of neutrophils on endothelium and consequently transendothelial neutrophil migration response to sites of infection. PECAM-1 is a phosphoprotein highly expressed on endothelial cells and leukocytes, and comprises an important component in the regulation of neutrophil transendothelial migration. Endocan is a proteoglycan expressed and secreted by the vascular endothelium in response to pro-inflammatory cytokines and pro-angiogenic factors, and inhibits leukocyte migration. The soluble forms of these proteins have been found increased in the sera of septic patients. uPAR is a part of the plasminogen activation system, which is involved in tissue reorganization events. The soluble form of uPAR, suPAR, forms when UPA binds to uPAR, and its levels are increased in sepsis. TREM-1 is an inflammatory immunoglobulin superfamily member, which is expressed in neutrophils, monocytes, and macrophages. TREM-1 triggers and expands the inflammatory response, with promoted production of inflammatory mediators, inhibited expression of anti-inflammatory mediators, and activated and amplified inflammatory cascade. sTREM-1 is a subtype of secreted TREM-1, which has been shown to be released into the blood during infection. The protein C anticoagulant system also involves protein S, and the endothelial receptors TM and EPCR. Conversion of protein C to the anticoagulant APC is generated by TM-bound thrombin and is drastically augmented by the presence of EPCR. The presence of a soluble form of EPCR (sEPCR) is elevated in conditions marked by enhanced inflammation, of unknown physiological significance. CD14 is yet another glycoprotein expressed on monocytes and macrophages, and serves as a receptor for lipopolysaccharides. As a pattern recognition molecule it plays a role in the innate immune system by activating a pro-inflammatory signaling cascade upon contact with microorganisms. During inflammation, protease activity releases soluble CD14 (sCD14) fragments, one of which has been identified as presepsin. Other pattern recognition receptors involved in immunity are TLRs. Stimulation of TLRs by microbial components triggers expression of several genes that are involved in immune responses. Finally, lactate is also increased due to production by various tissues through aerobic and anaerobic glycolysis, and from a decreased lactate clearance. Ang-1, angiopoietin-1; Ang-2, angiopoietin-2, APC, activated protein C; CD14, cluster of differentiation 14; CRP, C-reactive protein; IL, interleukin; PCT, procalcitonin; sEPCR, soluble endothelial protein C receptor; sICAM-1, soluble intercellular adhesion molecule-1; sPECAM-1, soluble platelet/endothelial cell adhesion molecule-1; sTREM-1, soluble triggering receptor expressed on myeloid cells-1; suPAR, soluble urokinase-type plasminogen activator receptor; TM, thrombomodulin; TNF-α, tumor necrosis factor-alpha; TLR, Toll-like receptors; UPA, urokinase-type plasminogen activator.

3. Genetic polymorphisms in sepsis

The prospective of genetic biomarkers for prognostic use is well-known for mostly uncommon/rare inherited disorders, but is also emerging for sepsis [185, 186]. Most genes carry single-nucleotide polymorphisms (SNPs) at specific exonic or intronic regions.

In order to identify potential markers of susceptibility, severity, and clinical outcome, potential markers for survivors and nonsurvivors, and ultimately to identify targets for therapeutic intervention, gene polymorphisms have become the most widely used form of experimental study. In an attempt to deal with the limitations of these studies, such as small sample size and bias in selecting candidate polymorphisms and genes, genome-wide association studies (GWAS) are now emerging. GWAS concern large, well-conducted, multicenter studies that do not involve a prior hypothesis of candidate genes to test for association with disease.

3.1. Cell signaling pathways of the innate immune system

3.1.1. Pattern recognition receptors (PRR)

3.1.1.1. Toll-like receptors (TLRs)

Functional characterization of Toll-like receptors (TLRs) has established that innate immunity is an adept system that detects invasion of microbial pathogens. Stimulation of TLRs by microbial components triggers expression of several genes that are involved in immune responses [187]. TLR4 is an essential receptor for Gram-negative enteric LPS recognition [188, 189]. The Asp299Gly mutation in human TLR4 impairs LPS signaling in homozygous and heterozygous individuals [190], while Smirnova *et al.* [191] observed that rare heterozygous missense mutations of TLR4 contribute to the development of systemic meningococcal disease. The D299G allele of the *TLR4* gene has also been associated with increased susceptibility to severe bacterial infections and Gram-negative sepsis [192, 193].

3.1.2. Cellular innate immune response

3.1.2.1. IL-8

The 251A/T allele (rs4073) of the *IL-8* gene has been studied for its implication in sepsis and outcomes. Results until now have shown association of the allele with higher plasma IL-8 levels, as well as with survival [194]. The A allele has been suggested to be associated with protection against sepsis [195], and also with increased risk of sepsis [196]. The heterozygote AT genotype has been associated with increased risk of developing severe sepsis [197]. In a more recent study, the male population carrying the homozygote TT genotype was found to be more susceptible to sepsis, while no association was determined between the 251A/T allele and IL-8 serum levels in septic patients [198].

3.2. Adaptive immune response

3.2.1. Cytokines

3.2.1.1. Tumor necrosis factor-α promoter polymorphisms

Initially, the G-to-A polymorphism at position 308nt in the promoter region of the *TNF-α* gene was found to be associated with adverse outcome in patients with severe sepsis and septic shock [199, 200]. A large meta-analysis [201] concluded that the polymorphism is associated with sepsis, but is not associated with sepsis mortality. However, several studies later were not able to show association of *TNF-α*-308 SNP and development of sepsis [202, 203].

3.2.1.2. IL-6 polymorphisms

A key inflammatory cytokine that has been examined in genetic association studies in infectious diseases is , producing also conflicting results. First of all, studies on the C allele of the G/C polymorphism at position 174nt of the IL-6 gene have shown its association with both high and low plasma IL-6 levels [204, 205], or even no association at all [206]. One study in critically ill patients did not find association between the 174 G/C polymorphism and sepsis appearance, but associated the polymorphism with improved survival rates in patients with sepsis [207]. A different study reported that the same polymorphism was not associated with survival [208]. A meta-analysis on the position 174nt polymorphism and the risk of sepsis in very low birth weight infants concluded that the available data are not consistent with more than a modest association between the *IL-6* polymorphism and neonatal sepsis [209].

3.3. Systemic effectors of inflammation and coagulation

3.3.1. Angiotensin-converting enzyme (ACE)

Studies have compared the effects of the angiotensin-converting enzyme (*ACE*) insertion/deletion (I/D) polymorphisms on the incidence and outcome of sepsis and acute respiratory distress syndrome (ARDS). In ventilated low birth weight infants the *ACE* insertion/deletion (I/D) polymorphism does not have a significant effect on the incidence or outcome of sepsis [210, 211]. Studies and meta-analyses showed that carriers of I allele (D/I genotype and I/I genotype) were at increased sepsis risk [212–214], but the polymorphism is not associated with outcome in critically ill septic patients [214, 215]. With regard to ARDS, the data of Villar *et al.* [216] do not support an association of the *ACE* gene I/D polymorphism with susceptibility or mortality in severe sepsis or with sepsis-induced ARDS in Spanish patients, but Cardinal-Fernandez *et al.* demonstrated that the presence of the allele D of the *ACE* gene is associated with ARDS in patients with severe sepsis [217].

3.3.2. *Endothelial protein C receptor (EPCR)*

A few studies have compared the effects of the *EPCR* haplotypes on the incidence and outcome of sepsis. Two studies have shown that *EPCR* mutations and polymorphisms influence the risk of severe sepsis in children and adults [218, 219]. More specifically, the rare 23-bp insertion is significantly more common among patients with severe sepsis [218], while simultaneous carriers of minor alleles belonging to both the H1 and H3 haplotypes may be at reduced risk of developing severe sepsis and/or septic shock among critically ill patients [219].

Table 1 lists the role of major circulating biomarkers and genetic polymorphisms in the prognosis and diagnosis of sepsis.

Biomarker	Diagnostic significance	Prognostic significance
C-reactive protein (CRP)	- Discriminates bacterial and viral infections [14]	- CRP is a valuable marker for the disease severity [15, 20]
	- Measurement of CRP is an indicator of sepsis [15–19]	- Elevated concentrations of serum CRP on admission have been associated with increased risk of organ failure and mortality [21, 22]
Procalcitonin (PCT)	- PCT is important in the detection and differential diagnosis of inflammatory states [26]. The highest levels of PCT are achieved in acute bacterial infections and sepsis	- PCT nonclearance is a prognostic factor of death in patients with sepsis [33]
	- PCT is a good biological diagnostic marker for sepsis, severe sepsis, or septic shock [34]	- Significant difference between PCT levels as early as day 1 between survivors and nonsurvivors among septic patients [37]
	- PCT is a helpful biomarker for early diagnosis of sepsis in critically ill patients [36]	
	- Serial PCT concentrations may have value in monitoring sepsis outcomes [28, 29]	
Tumor necrosis factor-α (TNF-α)	- Levels of TNF-α are frequently increased in sepsis [49, 56]	- High concentrations of TNF-α are predictive of organ failure and increased mortality in septic patients [55]
Interleukin-1β (IL-1β)	- Levels of IL-1β are frequently increased in sepsis [56]	
Interleukin-6 (IL-6)	- Levels of IL-6 are frequently increased in sepsis [50, 54, 56]	- High concentrations of IL-6 are predictive of organ failure and increased mortality in septic patients [57, 59]
	- IL-6 levels are increased in patients with infectious complications and have been used to differentiate systemic inflammatory response syndrome (SIRS) from sepsis [58]	

Biomarker	Diagnostic significance	Prognostic significance
Interleukin-8 (IL-8)	- Levels of IL-8 are frequently increased in sepsis [50, 56]	- IL-8 has been used to predict the severity of sepsis in pediatric patients, although the use of IL-8 has not been confirmed in adults [60, 61]
Interleukin-27 (IL-27)	- Useful biomarker in estimating risk of bacterial infection among critically ill pediatric and adult patients [67–70] - In combination with PCT, IL-27 may improve classification of critically ill adults with sepsis [68, 71]	
Interleukin-10 (IL-10)		- Poor patient outcome has been associated with increased blood levels of the anti-inflammatory cytokine IL-10 [74]
Angiopoietin-1 (Ang-1)	- Decreased levels in critically ill septic or nonseptic patients compared to healthy controls [94]	- Decreased levels of Ang-1 at ICU admission are correlated with higher mortality [97]
Angiopoietin-2 (Ang-2)	- Ang-2 levels are higher in patients with severe sepsis compared to patients with or without SIRS or sepsis [89–91]	- Increased Ang-2 plasma levels have been associated with worst clinical outcome in patients with major trauma and severe sepsis or shock [92–94] - Increased Ang-2 plasma in nonsurvivors compared to survivors [95, 96]
Selectins	- Soluble E-selectin concentration increases in various inflammatory pathologies [99–102]	- Higher sE-selectin levels in nonsurvivors than survivors [103, 104] - sE-selectin levels may be used as predictor of fatal outcome in patients with SIRS [105] - sE-selectin has also been proposed as a predictor of bacteremia in severe sepsis patients [106] High levels of sE- and sP-selectin at ICU admission, are associated with sepsis development in time [109]
Soluble in tercellular adhesion molecule-1 (sICAM-1)	-s ICAM-1 production has been shown to be related to increased sepsis severity [102, 111] - sICAM-1 appears to be a reliable biomarker for classifying patients with infectious SIRS, i.e., sepsis, from those with noninfectious SIRS [105]	- sICAM-1 concentration has been shown to be related to increased mortality [111, 112]
Soluble platelet/endothelial cell adhesion molecule-1 (sPECAM-1)	- sPECAM-1 is higher at admission in septic patients compared with nonseptic patients and healthy controls [114, 115]	
Endocan	- Exhibits higher concentrations in septic patients compared to healthy volunteers [117]	- A strong and significant predictor of sepsis severity and outcome [118–122]

Biomarker	Diagnostic significance	Prognostic significance
Soluble urokinase-type plasminogen activator receptor (suPAR)	- Elevated suPAR in conditions of SIRS, bacteremia, sepsis, and septic shock [124–127]	- High circulating suPAR levels indicate an unfavorable prognosis, including organ dysfunction and mortality [124–127]
	- Diagnostic value of suPAR for identifying sepsis is limited [128]	- In patients with bacteremia, suPAR may be used to identify severely ill patients and predict mortality [131, 133]
Soluble triggering receptor expressed on myeloid cells-1 (sTREM-1)	- Moderate diagnostic performance in differentiating sepsis from SIRS [140]	- Moderate prognostic significance in assessing the mortality of infection in adult patients and sTREM-1 alone is insufficient to predict mortality as a biomarker [142]
	- sTREM-1 represents a reliable biological marker of bacterial infection [143]	
Soluble endothelial protein C receptor (sEPCR)	- sEPCR levels in septic patients have been found to be significantly higher [146, 147], unchanged [148], or lower [149] than in healthy volunteers	- sEPCR levels correlated with worst outcomes; has been suggested that it may act as a biological marker of outcome in severe sepsis [150–152]
		- Levels of sEPCR at ICU admission are higher in originally nonseptic patients who subsequently become septic compared to those who will not [152]
Presepsin	- Discriminates between bacterial and nonbacterial infections [155]	- Initial values significantly correlated with in-hospital mortality of patients affected by sepsis, severe sepsis, or septic shock [156]
	- Early diagnosis of infection in a population of patients with SIRS, sepsis, severe sepsis, and septic shock [153]	- Presepsin reveals prognostic value with respect to 30 days and 6 months all-cause mortality throughout the first week of ICU treatment [153]
	- In patients with suspected severe sepsis and septic shock, presepsin reveals valuable diagnostic capacity to differentiate sepsis severity [156]	- Presepsin measured on the first day in ICU in patients with severe sepsis or septic shock was higher in nonsurvivors compared to survivors [157]
	- Presepsin can differentiate between septic and nonseptic patients with comparable accuracy to CRP and PCT [161, 162]	
Lactate	- Elevated serum lactate levels in sepsis [177, 178]	- Elevated serum lactate levels are associated with poor outcomes in diverse populations of critically ill patients, such as multiple organ failure, morbidity, and mortality [172–175]
	- Early serum lactate levels can diagnose sepsis in undifferentiated patients with suspected sepsis [176, 179]	- Serum lactate is a potentially useful biomarker to risk-stratify patients with severe sepsis presenting to the emergency department [170, 174, 175]

Biomarker	Diagnostic significance	Prognostic significance
		- Combining sE- and sP-selectin with serum lactate offers better prognostic value for sepsis development in initially nonseptic ICU patients [180]
Genetic polymorphisms	- Distinguish patients with sepsis from patients with sterile inflammation	- Predict long-term outcomes and identify patients who will be at risk for developing adverse clinical outcomes
Toll-like receptors (TLRs)		- D299G allele of *TLR4* gene associated with increased susceptibility to severe bacterial infections and Gram-negative sepsis [192, 193]
IL-8		- The 251A/T allele has been associated with survival [194], protection against sepsis [195], and also increased risk of sepsis [196]
		- The heterozygote AT genotype has been associated with increased risk of developing sepsis [197]
		- Male T allele carriers are more susceptible to sepsis [198]
TNF-α	- G-to-A polymorphism associated with sepsis [201]	- G-to-A polymorphism associated with adverse outcomes in patients with severe sepsis and septic shock [199, 200]
	- No association of G-to-A polymorphism and development of sepsis [202, 203]	- G-to-A polymorphism not associated with sepsis mortality [201]
IL-6	- 174 G/C polymorphism showed modest association with neonatal sepsis [209]	- 174 G/C polymorphism was associated with improved survival rates in patients with sepsis [207]
		- 174 G/C polymorphism was not associated with a difference in survival [208]
Angiotensin-converting enzyme (*ACE*)		- Insertion/deletion (I/D) polymorphism does not have an effect on the incidence or outcome of sepsis in ventilated low birth infants [210, 211]
		- Carriers of the I allele at increased sepsis risk [212–214]
		- I polymorphism not associated with outcome in critically ill septic patients [214–216]
		- The presence of the D allele is associated with ARDS in patients with severe sepsis [217]

Biomarker	Diagnostic significance	Prognostic significance
Endothelial protein C receptor (*EPCR*)	- The rare 23-bp insertion is significantly more common among patients with severe sepsis [218]	- Influences the risk of severe sepsis in children and adults [218, 219]
		- Simultaneous carriers of minor alleles belonging to both the H1 and H3 haplotypes may be at reduced risk of developing severe sepsis and/or septic shock among critically ill patients [219]

Table 1. Role of major circulating biomarkers and genetic polymorphisms in sepsis. Please note that the protein names are capitalized, whereas gene names are capitalized and italicized.

4. Conclusion

Unfortunately, a lot of work remains to find the right combination of markers to be used in clinical practice. Some have been effective in reducing mortality, but their use in diagnosis and prognosis of sepsis has been limited. It seems that a panel of diverse biomarkers rather than a group of two or three related biomarkers will be more efficient in clinical practice.

Genome-wide association studies may help confirm current findings and make them clinically applicable. Hence, developing high-throughput approaches for the analysis of alternative mechanisms by which SNPs can cause disease will be one of the remaining challenges for genomic research. Hopefully, the findings that will be generated will facilitate the successful use of modern molecular diagnostics and could enable rapid identification of particularly susceptible or less susceptible individuals, leading to tailored therapeutic approaches.

Acknowledgements

The authors would like to thank Mr. Antonis Makriyannis for his excellent artwork (**Figure 1**).

Author details

Alice Georgia Vassiliou[1*], Stylianos E. Orfanos[1,3] and Anastasia Kotanidou[1,2]

*Address all correspondence to: alvass75@gmail.com

1 First Department of Critical Care Medicine & Pulmonary Services, GP Livanos and M Simou Laboratories, National and Kapodistrian University of Athens Medical School, Evangelismos Hospital, Athens, Greece

2 First Department of Critical Care Medicine & Pulmonary Services, National and Kapodistrian University of Athens Medical School, Evangelismos Hospital, Athens, Greece

3 Second Department of Critical Care, National and Kapodistrian University of Athens Medical School, Attikon Hospital, Athens, Greece

References

[1] Singer M, Deutschman CS, Seymour CW, Shankar-Hari M, Annane D, Bauer M, et al. The Third International Consensus Definitions for Sepsis and Septic Shock (Sepsis-3). The Journal of the American Medical Association. 2016 Feb 23;315(8):801-10.

[2] Levy MM, Fink MP, Marshall JC, Abraham E, Angus D, Cook D, et al. 2001 SCCM/ESICM/ACCP/ATS/SIS International Sepsis Definitions Conference. Intensive Care Medicine. 2003 Apr;29(4):530-8.

[3] Angus DC, van der Poll T. Severe sepsis and septic shock. The New England Journal of Medicine. 2013 Aug 29;369(9):840-51.

[4] Rhodes A, Evans LE, Alhazzani W, Levy MM, Antonelli M, Ferrer R, et al. Surviving Sepsis Campaign: International guidelines for management of sepsis and septic shock: 2016. Critical Care Medicine. 2017 Mar;45(3):486-552.

[5] Dellinger RP, Levy MM, Rhodes A, Annane D, Gerlach H, Opal SM, et al. Surviving Sepsis Campaign: International guidelines for management of severe sepsis and septic shock, 2012. Intensive Care Medicine. 2013 Feb;39(2):165-228.

[6] Levy MM, Dellinger RP, Townsend SR, Linde-Zwirble WT, Marshall JC, Bion J, et al. The surviving sepsis campaign: Results of an international guideline-based performance improvement program targeting severe sepsis. Intensive Care Medicine. 2010 Feb;36(2):222-31.

[7] Vincent JL, Opal SM, Marshall JC, Tracey KJ. Sepsis definitions: Time for change. Lancet. 2013 Mar 2;381(9868):774-5.

[8] Deutschman CS, Tracey KJ. Sepsis: Current dogma and new perspectives. Immunity. 2014 Apr 17;40(4):463-75.

[9] Angus DC. Drotrecogin alfa (activated)…a sad final fizzle to a roller-coaster party. Critical Care. 2012 Feb 06;16(1):107.

[10] Hotchkiss RS, Monneret G, Payen D. Sepsis-induced immunosuppression: From cellular dysfunctions to immunotherapy. Nature Reviews Immunology. 2013 Dec;13(12):862-74.

[11] Singer M, De Santis V, Vitale D, Jeffcoate W. Multiorgan failure is an adaptive, endocrine-mediated, metabolic response to overwhelming systemic inflammation. Lancet. 2004 Aug 7-13;364(9433):545-8.

[12] Vincent JL, Beumier M. Diagnostic and prognostic markers in sepsis: Expert review of anti-infective therapy. 2013 Mar;11(3):265-75.

[13] Pepys MB, Hirschfield GM. C-reactive protein: A critical update. Journal of Clinical Investigation. 2003 Jun;111(12):1805-12.

[14] Shaw AC. Serum C-reactive protein and neopterin concentrations in patients with viral or bacterial infection. Journal of Clinical Pathology. 1991 Jul;44(7):596-9.

[15] Ugarte H, Silva E, Mercan D, De Mendonca A, Vincent JL. Procalcitonin used as a marker of infection in the intensive care unit. Critical Care Medicine. 1999 Mar;27(3):498-504.

[16] Huntley JS, Kelly MB. C-reactive protein: A valuable acute investigation: A case of pneumococcal meningitis presenting as ankle pain. Emergency Medicine Journal. 2005 Aug;22(8):602-3.

[17] Kawczynski P, Piotrowski A. Procalcitonin and C-reactive protein as a markers of neonatal sepsis. Ginekologia Polska. 2004 Jun;75(6):439-44.

[18] Povoa P. C-reactive protein: A valuable marker of sepsis. Intensive Care Medicine. 2002 Mar;28(3):235-43.

[19] Povoa P, Teixeira-Pinto AM, Carneiro AH. C-reactive protein, an early marker of community-acquired sepsis resolution: A multi-center prospective observational study. Critical Care. 2011 Jul 15;15(4):R169.

[20] Suprin E, Camus C, Gacouin A, Le Tulzo Y, Lavoue S, Feuillu A, et al. Procalcitonin: A valuable indicator of infection in a medical ICU? Intensive Care Medicine. 2000 Sep;26(9):1232-8.

[21] Devran O, Karakurt Z, Adiguzel N, Gungor G, Mocin OY, Balci MK, et al. C-reactive protein as a predictor of mortality in patients affected with severe sepsis in intensive care unit. Multidisciplinary Respiratory Medicine. 2012 Nov 21;7(1):47.

[22] Lobo SM, Lobo FR, Bota DP, Lopes-Ferreira F, Soliman HM, Melot C, et al. C-reactive protein levels correlate with mortality and organ failure in critically ill patients. Chest. 2003 Jun;123(6):2043-9.

[23] Miguel-Bayarri V, Casanoves-Laparra EB, Pallas-Beneyto L, Sancho-Chinesta S, Martin-Osorio LF, Tormo-Calandin C, et al. Prognostic value of the biomarkers procalcitonin, interleukin-6 and C-reactive protein in severe sepsis. Medicina Intensiva. 2012 Nov;36(8):556-62.

[24] Tschaikowsky K, Hedwig-Geissing M, Braun GG, Radespiel-Troeger M. Predictive value of procalcitonin, interleukin-6, and C-reactive protein for survival in postoperative patients with severe sepsis. Journal of Critical Care. 2011 Feb;26(1):54-64.

[25] Maruna P, Nedelnikova K, Gurlich R. Physiology and genetics of procalcitonin. Physiological Research. 2000;49(Suppl. 1):S57-61.

[26] Assicot M, Gendrel D, Carsin H, Raymond J, Guilbaud J, Bohuon C. High serum procalcitonin concentrations in patients with sepsis and infection. Lancet. 1993 Feb 27;341 (8844):515-8.

[27] Reinhart K, Bauer M, Riedemann NC, Hartog CS. New approaches to sepsis: Molecular diagnostics and biomarkers. Clinical Microbiology Reviews. 2012 Oct;25(4):609-34. PubMed PMID: 23034322. Pubmed Central PMCID: PMC3485751. Epub 2012/10/05. Eng.

[28] de Azevedo JR, Torres OJ, Beraldi RA, Ribas CA, Malafaia O. Prognostic evaluation of severe sepsis and septic shock: Procalcitonin clearance vs delta sequential organ failure assessment. Journal of Critical Care. 2015 Feb;30(1):219 e9-12.

[29] Sridharan P, Chamberlain RS. The efficacy of procalcitonin as a biomarker in the management of sepsis: Slaying dragons or tilting at windmills? Surgical Infections. 2013 Dec;14(6):489-511.

[30] Huang MY, Chen CY, Chien JH, Wu KH, Chang YJ, Wu KH, et al. Serum procalcitonin and procalcitonin clearance as a prognostic biomarker in patients with severe sepsis and septic shock. Biomed Research International. 2016;2016:1758501.

[31] Mat Nor MB, Md Ralib A. Procalcitonin clearance for early prediction of survival in critically ill patients with severe sepsis. Critical Care Research and Practice. 2014;2014:819034. PubMed PMID: 24719759.

[32] Shi Y, Peng JM, Hu XY, Wang Y. The utility of initial procalcitonin and procalcitonin clearance for prediction of bacterial infection and outcome in critically ill patients with autoimmune diseases: A prospective observational study. BMC Anesthesiology. 2015 Oct 07;15:137.

[33] Liu D, Su L, Han G, Yan P, Xie L. Prognostic value of procalcitonin in adult patients with sepsis: A systematic review and meta-analysis. PLoS One. 2015;10(6):e0129450. PubMed PMID: 26076027.

[34] Uzzan B, Cohen R, Nicolas P, Cucherat M, Perret GY. Procalcitonin as a diagnostic test for sepsis in critically ill adults and after surgery or trauma: A systematic review and meta-analysis. Critical Care Medicine. 2006 Jul;34(7):1996-2003.

[35] Tang BM, Eslick GD, Craig JC, McLean AS. Accuracy of procalcitonin for sepsis diagnosis in critically ill patients: Systematic review and meta-analysis. The Lancet Infectious Diseases. 2007 Mar;7(3):210-7.

[36] Wacker C, Prkno A, Brunkhorst FM, Schlattmann P. Procalcitonin as a diagnostic marker for sepsis: A systematic review and meta-analysis. The Lancet Infectious Diseases. 2013 May;13(5):426-35.

[37] Arora S, Singh P, Singh PM, Trikha A. Procalcitonin levels in survivors and nonsurvivors of sepsis: Systematic review and meta-analysis. Shock. 2015 Mar;43(3):212-21.

[38] Prkno A, Wacker C, Brunkhorst FM, Schlattmann P. Procalcitonin-guided therapy in intensive care unit patients with severe sepsis and septic shock: A systematic review and meta-analysis. Critical Care. 2013;17(6):R291.

[39] Oberhoffer M, Vogelsang H, Russwurm S, Hartung T, Reinhart K. Outcome prediction by traditional and new markers of inflammation in patients with sepsis. Clinical Chemistry and Laboratory Medicine. 1999 Mar;37(3):363-8.

[40] Schroder J, Staubach KH, Zabel P, Stuber F, Kremer B. Procalcitonin as a marker of severity in septic shock. Langenbeck's Archives of Surgery. 1999 Feb;384(1):33-8.

[41] Nargis W, Ibrahim M, Ahamed BU. Procalcitonin versus C-reactive protein: Usefulness as biomarker of sepsis in ICU patient. International Journal of Critical Illness and Injury Science. 2014 Jul;4(3):195-9.

[42] Selberg O, Hecker H, Martin M, Klos A, Bautsch W, Kohl J. Discrimination of sepsis and systemic inflammatory response syndrome by determination of circulating plasma concentrations of procalcitonin, protein complement 3a, and interleukin-6. Critical Care Medicine. 2000 Aug;28(8):2793-8.

[43] Simon L, Gauvin F, Amre D, Saint-Louis P, Lacroix J. Serum procalcitonin and C-reactive protein levels as markers of bacterial infection: A systematic review and meta-analysis. Clinical Infectious Diseases. 2004;39(2):206-17.

[44] Bone RC. Sir Isaac Newton, sepsis, SIRS, and CARS. Critical Care Medicine. 1996;24(7):1 125-8.

[45] Tamayo E, Fernández A, Almansa R, Carrasco E, Heredia M, Lajo C, et al. Pro- and anti-inflammatory responses are regulated simultaneously from the first moments of septic shock. European Cytokine Network. 2011;22:82-7.

[46] Sherwin C, Broadbent R, Young S, Worth J, McCaffrey F, Medlicott NJ, et al. Utility of interleukin-12 and interleukin-10 in comparison with other cytokines and acute-phase reactants in the diagnosis of neonatal sepsis. The American Journal of Perinatology. 2008;25:629-36.

[47] Engel A, Mack E, Kern P, Kern W. An analysis of interleukin-8, interleukin-6 and C-reactive protein serum concentrations to predict fever, gram-negative bacteremia and complicated infection in neutropenic cancer patients. Infection. 1998;26:213-21.

[48] Kolaczkowska E, Kubes P. Neutrophil recruitment and function in health and inflammation. Nature Reviews Immunology. 2013 Mar;13(3):159-75.

[49] Lewis SM, Treacher DF, Bergmeier L, Brain SD, Chambers DJ, Pearson JD, et al. Plasma from patients with sepsis up-regulates the expression of CD49d and CD64 on blood neutrophils. The American Journal of Respiratory Cell and Molecular Biology. 2009 Jun;40(6):724-32.

[50] Harbarth S, Holeckova K, Froidevaux C, Pittet D, Ricou B, Grau GE, et al. Diagnostic value of procalcitonin, interleukin-6, and interleukin-8 in critically ill patients admitted with suspected sepsis. The American Journal of Respiratory and Critical Care Medicine. 2001 Aug 1;164(3):396-402.

[51] Bosmann M, Ward PA. Therapeutic potential of targeting IL-17 and IL-23 in sepsis. Clinical and Translational Medicine. 2012;1(1):4.

[52] Tschoeke SK, Oberholzer A, Moldawer LL. Interleukin-18: A novel prognostic cytokine in bacteria-induced sepsis. Critical Care Medicine. 2006 Apr;34(4):1225-33.

[53] Bingold TM, Ziesche E, Scheller B, Sadik CD, Franck K, Just L, et al. Interleukin-22 detected in patients with abdominal sepsis. Shock. 2010 Oct;34(4):337-40.

[54] Calandra T, Gerain J, Heumann D, Baumgartner JD, Glauser MP. High circulating levels of interleukin-6 in patients with septic shock: Evolution during sepsis, prognostic value, and interplay with other cytokines. The Swiss-Dutch J5 Immunoglobulin Study Group. The American Journal of Medicine. 1991 Jul;91(1):23-9.

[55] Damas P, Reuter A, Gysen P, Demonty J, Lamy M, Franchimont P. Tumor necrosis factor and interleukin-1 serum levels during severe sepsis in humans. Critical Care Medicine. 1989 Oct;17(10):975-8.

[56] Kurt AN, Aygun AD, Godekmerdan A, Kurt A, Dogan Y, Yilmaz E. Serum IL-1beta, IL-6, IL-8, and TNF-alpha levels in early diagnosis and management of neonatal sepsis. Mediators of Inflammation. 2007;2007:31397.

[57] Pettila V, Hynninen M, Takkunen O, Kuusela P, Valtonen M. Predictive value of procalcitonin and interleukin 6 in critically ill patients with suspected sepsis. Intensive Care Medicine. 2002 Sep;28(9):1220-5.

[58] Du B, Pan J, Chen D, Li Y. Serum procalcitonin and interleukin-6 levels may help to differentiate systemic inflammatory response of infectious and non-infectious origin. Chinese Medical Journal. 2003 Apr;116(4):538-42.

[59] Kellum JA, Kong L, Fink MP, Weissfeld LA, Yealy DM, Pinsky MR, et al. Understanding the inflammatory cytokine response in pneumonia and sepsis: Results of the genetic and inflammatory markers of sepsis (GenIMS) study. Archives of Internal Medicine. 2007 Aug 13-27;167(15):1655-63.

[60] Calfee CS, Thompson BT, Parsons PE, Ware LB, Matthay MA, Wong HR. Plasma interleukin-8 is not an effective risk stratification tool for adults with vasopressor-dependent septic shock. Critical Care Medicine. 2010 Jun;38(6):1436-41.

[61] Wong HR, Cvijanovich N, Wheeler DS, Bigham MT, Monaco M, Odoms K, et al. Interleukin-8 as a stratification tool for interventional trials involving pediatric septic shock. The American Journal of Respiratory and Critical Care Medicine. 2008 Aug 1;178(3):276-82.

[62] Lang Y, Jiang Y, Gao M, Wang W, Wang N, Wang K, et al. Interleukin-1 Receptor 2: A new biomarker for sepsis diagnosis and gram-negative/gram-positive bacterial differentiation. Shock. 2017 Jan;47(1):119-24.

[63] Abraham E, Anzueto A, Gutierrez G, Tessler S, San Pedro G, Wunderink R, et al. Double-blind randomised controlled trial of monoclonal antibody to human tumour necrosis factor in treatment of septic shock. NORASEPT II Study Group. Lancet. 1998 Mar 28;351(9107):929-33.

[64] van der Poll T, Levi M, Hack CE, ten Cate H, van Deventer SJ, Eerenberg AJ, et al. wElimination of interleukin 6 attenuates coagulation activation in experimental endotoxemia in chimpanzees. Journal of Experimental Medicine. 1994 Apr 1;179(4):1253-9.

[65] Boermeester MA, van Leeuwen PA, Coyle SM, Wolbink GJ, Hack CE, Lowry SF. Interleukin-1 blockade attenuates mediator release and dysregulation of the hemostatic mechanism during human sepsis. Archives of Surgery (Chicago, IL: 1960). 1995 Jul;130(7):739-48.

[66] Brown KA, Brown GA, Lewis SM, Beale R, Treacher DF. Targeting cytokines as a treatment for patients with sepsis: A lost cause or a strategy still worthy of pursuit? International Immunopharmacology. 2016 Jul;36:291-9.

[67] Wong HR, Cvijanovich NZ, Hall M, Allen GL, Thomas NJ, Freishtat RJ, et al. Interleukin-27 is a novel candidate diagnostic biomarker for bacterial infection in critically ill children. Critical Care. 2012 Oct 29;16(5):R213.

[68] Wong HR, Lindsell CJ, Lahni P, Hart KW, Gibot S. Interleukin 27 as a sepsis diagnostic biomarker in critically ill adults. Shock. 2013 Nov;40(5):382-6.

[69] Wong HR, Liu KD, Kangelaris KN, Lahni P, Calfee CS. Performance of interleukin-27 as a sepsis diagnostic biomarker in critically ill adults. Journal of Critical Care. 2014 Oct;29(5):718-22.

[70] Hanna WJ, Berrens Z, Langner T, Lahni P, Wong HR. Interleukin-27: A novel biomarker in predicting bacterial infection among the critically ill. Critical Care. 2015 Oct 30;19:378.

[71] Fu J, Wang Y, Zeng P, Niu S. Value of interleukin-27 as a diagnostic biomarker of sepsis in critically ill adults. Zhonghua wei zhong bing ji jiu yi xue. 2015 Jun;27(6):460-4.

[72] Ward N, Casserly B, Ayala A. The compensatory anti-inflammatory response syndrome (CARS) in critically ill patients. Clinics in Chest Medicine. 2008;29(4):617-25.

[73] Oberholzer A, Oberholzer C, Moldawer L. Interleukin-10: A complex role in the pathogenesis of sepsis syndromes and its potential as an anti-inflammatory drug. Critical Care Medicine. 2002;30(1 Suppl.):S58-63.

[74] Monneret G, Finck ME, Venet F, Debard AL, Bohe J, Bienvenu J, et al. The anti-inflammatory response dominates after septic shock: Association of low monocyte HLA-DR expression and high interleukin-10 concentration. Immunology Letters. 2004 Sep;95(2):193-8.

[75] Berg D, Kühn R, Rajewsky K, Müller W, Menon S, Davidson N, et al. Interleukin-10 is a central regulator of the response to LPS in murine models of endotoxic shock and the Shwartzman reaction but not endotoxin tolerance. The Journal of Clinical Investigation. 1995;96(5):2339-47.

[76] Howard M, Muchamuel T, Andrade S, Menon S. Interleukin 10 protects mice from lethal endotoxemia. Journal of Experimental Medicine. 1993;177(4):1205-8.

[77] van der Poll T, Jansen P, Montegut W, Braxton C, Calvano S, Stackpole S, et al. Effects of IL-10 on systemic inflammatory responses during sublethal primate endotoxemia. Journal of Immunology. 1997;158(4):1971-5.

[78] Remick D, Garg S, Newcomb D, Wollenberg G, Huie T, Bolgos G. Exogenous interleukin-10 fails to decrease the mortality or morbidity of sepsis. Critical Care Medicine. 1998;26(5):985-04.

[79] Steinhauser M, Hogaboam C, Kunkel S, Lukacs N, Strieter R, Standiford T. IL-10 is a major mediator of sepsis-induced impairment in lung antibacterial host defense. Journal of Immunology. 1999;162(1):392-9.

[80] Song G, Chung C, Chaudry I, Ayala A. What is the role of interleukin 10 in polymicrobial sepsis: Anti-inflammatory agent or immunosuppressant? Surgery. 1999;126(2):378-83.

[81] Ashare A, Powers L, Butler N, Doerschug K, Monick M, Hunninghake G. Anti-inflammatory response is associated with mortality and severity of infection in sepsis. The American Journal of Physiology – Lung Cellular and Molecular Physiology. 2005 ;288(4):L633-40.

[82] Panacek E, Marshall J, Albertson T, Johnson D, Johnson S, MacArthur R, et al. Efficacy and safety of the monoclonal anti-tumor necrosis factor antibody F(ab')2 fragment afelimomab in patients with severe sepsis and elevated interleukin-6 levels. Critical Care Medicine. 2004;32:2173-218.

[83] Maniatis NA, Kotanidou A, Catravas JD, Orfanos SE. Endothelial pathomechanisms in acute lung injury. Vascular Pharmacology. 2008 Oct–Dec;49(4-6):119-33.

[84] Maisonpierre PC, Suri C, Jones PF, Bartunkova S, Wiegand SJ, Radziejewski C, et al. Angiopoietin-2, a natural antagonist for Tie2 that disrupts in vivo angiogenesis. Science. 1997 Jul 4;277(5322):55-60.

[85] Thurston G, Rudge JS, Ioffe E, Zhou H, Ross L, Croll SD, et al. Angiopoietin-1 protects the adult vasculature against plasma leakage. Nature Medicine. 2000 Apr;6(4):460-3.

[86] Fiedler U, Augustin HG. Angiopoietins: A link between angiogenesis and inflammation. Trends Immunology. 2006 Dec;27(12):552-8.

[87] Roviezzo F, Tsigkos S, Kotanidou A, Bucci M, Brancaleone V, Cirino G, et al. Angiopoietin-2 causes inflammation in vivo by promoting vascular leakage. Journal of Pharmacology and Experimental Therapeutics. 2005 Aug;314(2):738-44.

[88] Xing K, Murthy S, Liles WC, Singh JM. Clinical utility of biomarkers of endothelial activation in sepsis – A systematic review. Critical Care. 2012;16(1):R7.

[89] Davis JS, Yeo TW, Piera KA, Woodberry T, Celermajer DS, Stephens DP, et al. Angiopoietin-2 is increased in sepsis and inversely associated with nitric oxide-dependent microvascular reactivity. Critical Care. 2010;14(3):R89.

[90] Orfanos SE, Kotanidou A, Glynos C, Athanasiou C, Tsigkos S, Dimopoulou I, et al. Angiopoietin-2 is increased in severe sepsis: Correlation with inflammatory mediators. Critical Care Medicine. 2007 Jan;35(1):199-206.

[91] Parikh SM, Mammoto T, Schultz A, Yuan HT, Christiani D, Karumanchi SA, et al. Excess circulating angiopoietin-2 may contribute to pulmonary vascular leak in sepsis in humans. PLoS Medicine. 2006 Mar;3(3):e46.

[92] Calfee CS, Gallagher D, Abbott J, Thompson BT, Matthay MA. Plasma angiopoietin-2 in clinical acute lung injury: Prognostic and pathogenetic significance. Critical Care Medicine. 2012 Jun;40(6):1731-7.

[93] Ganter MT, Cohen MJ, Brohi K, Chesebro BB, Staudenmayer KL, Rahn P, et al. Angiopoietin-2, marker and mediator of endothelial activation with prognostic significance early after trauma? Annals of Surgery. 2008 Feb;247(2):320-6.

[94] Ricciuto DR, dos Santos CC, Hawkes M, Toltl LJ, Conroy AL, Rajwans N, et al. Angiopoietin-1 and angiopoietin-2 as clinically informative prognostic biomarkers of morbidity and mortality in severe sepsis. Critical Care Medicine. 2011 Apr;39(4):702-10.

[95] Kranidioti H, Orfanos SE, Vaki I, Kotanidou A, Raftogiannis M, Dimopoulou I, et al. Angiopoietin-2 is increased in septic shock: Evidence for the existence of a circulating factor stimulating its release from human monocytes. Immunology Letters. 2009 Jun 30;125(1):65-71.

[96] Kumpers P, Lukasz A, David S, Horn R, Hafer C, Faulhaber-Walter R, et al. Excess circulating angiopoietin-2 is a strong predictor of mortality in critically ill medical patients. Critical Care. 2008;12(6):R147.

[97] Kumpers P, van Meurs M, David S, Molema G, Bijzet J, Lukasz A, et al. Time course of angiopoietin-2 release during experimental human endotoxemia and sepsis. Critical Care. 2009;13(3):R64.

[98] Tedder TF, Steeber DA, Chen A, Engel P. The selectins: Vascular adhesion molecules. FASEB Journal. 1995 Jul;9(10):866-73.

[99] Boldt J, Wollbruck M, Kuhn D, Linke LC, Hempelmann G. Do plasma levels of circulating soluble adhesion molecules differ between surviving and nonsurviving critically ill patients? Chest. 1995 Mar;107(3):787-92.

[100] Cowley HC, Heney D, Gearing AJ, Hemingway I, Webster NR. Increased circulating adhesion molecule concentrations in patients with the systemic inflammatory response syndrome: A prospective cohort study. Critical Care Medicine. 1994 Apr;22(4):651-7.

[101] Knapp S, Thalhammer F, Locker GJ, Laczika K, Hollenstein U, Frass M, et al. Prognostic value of MIP-1 alpha, TGF-beta 2, sELAM-1, and sVCAM-1 in patients with gram-positive sepsis. Clinical Immunology and Immunopathology. 1998 May;87(2):139-44.

[102] Sessler CN, Windsor AC, Schwartz M, Watson L, Fisher BJ, Sugerman HJ, et al. Circulating ICAM-1 is increased in septic shock. The American Journal of Respiratory and Critical Care Medicine. 1995 May;151(5):1420-7.

[103] Cummings CJ, Sessler CN, Beall LD, Fisher BJ, Best AM, Fowler AA, 3rd. Soluble E-selectin levels in sepsis and critical illness. Correlation with infection and

hemodynamic dysfunction. The American Journal of Respiratory and Critical Care Medicine. 1997 Aug;156(2 Pt 1):431-7.

[104] Simons RK, Hoyt DB, Winchell RJ, Rose RM, Holbrook T. Elevated selectin levels after severe trauma: A marker for sepsis and organ failure and a potential target for immunomodulatory therapy. Journal of Trauma. 1996 Oct;41(4):653-62.

[105] de Pablo R, Monserrat J, Reyes E, Diaz D, Rodriguez-Zapata M, de la Hera A, et al. Circulating sICAM-1 and sE-Selectin as biomarker of infection and prognosis in patients with systemic inflammatory response syndrome. European Journal of Internal Medicine. 2013 Mar; 24(2):132-8.

[106] Kung CT, Hsiao SY, Su CM, Tsai TC, Cheng HH, Tsai NW, et al. Serum adhesion molecules as predictors of bacteremia in adult severe sepsis patients at the emergency department. Clinica Chimica Acta. 2013 Feb 28;421:116-20.

[107] Sakamaki F, Ishizaka A, Handa M, Fujishima S, Urano T, Sayama K, et al. Soluble form of P-selectin in plasma is elevated in acute lung injury. The American Journal of Respiratory and Critical Care Medicine. 1995 Jun;151(6):1821-6.

[108] Wang HE, Shapiro NI, Griffin R, Safford MM, Judd S, Howard G. Inflammatory and endothelial activation biomarkers and risk of sepsis: A nested case–control study. Journal of Critical Care. 2013 Feb 12;28(5):549-55.

[109] Vassiliou AG, Mastora Z, Orfanos SE, Jahaj E, Maniatis NA, Koutsoukou A, et al. Elevated biomarkers of endothelial dysfunction/activation at ICU admission are associated with sepsis development. Cytokine. 2014 Jul 9;69(2):240-7.

[110] Muller WA. Leukocyte-endothelial-cell interactions in leukocyte transmigration and the inflammatory response. Trends in Immunology. 2003 Jun;24(6):327-34.

[111] Shapiro NI, Schuetz P, Yano K, Sorasaki M, Parikh SM, Jones AE, et al. The association of endothelial cell signaling, severity of illness, and organ dysfunction in sepsis. Critical Care. 2010;14(5):R182.

[112] Kayal S, Jais JP, Aguini N, Chaudiere J, Labrousse J. Elevated circulating E-selectin, intercellular adhesion molecule 1, and von Willebrand factor in patients with severe infection. The American Journal of Respiratory and Critical Care Medicine. 1998 Mar;157(3 Pt 1):776-84.

[113] Berman ME, Muller WA. Ligation of platelet/endothelial cell adhesion molecule 1 (PECAM-1/CD31) on monocytes and neutrophils increases binding capacity of leukocyte CR3 (CD11b/CD18). Journal of Immunology. 1995 Jan 01;154(1):299-307.

[114] Kjaergaard AG, Dige A, Nielsen JS, Tonnesen E, Krog J. The use of the soluble adhesion molecules sE-selectin, sICAM-1, sVCAM-1, sPECAM-1 and their ligands CD11a and CD49d as diagnostic and prognostic biomarkers in septic and critically ill non-septic ICU patients. Acta Pathologica, Microbiologica, et Immunologica Scandinavica. 2016 Oct;124(10):846-55.

[115] Sun W, Li FS, Zhang YH, Wang XP, Wang CR. Association of susceptibility to septic shock with platelet endothelial cell adhesion molecule-1 gene Leu125Val polymorphism and serum sPECAM-1 levels in sepsis patients. International Journal of Clinical and Experimental Medicine. 2015;8(11):20490-8.

[116] Bechard D, Gentina T, Delehedde M, Scherpereel A, Lyon M, Aumercier M, et al. Endocan is a novel chondroitin sulfate/dermatan sulfate proteoglycan that promotes hepatocyte growth factor/scatter factor mitogenic activity. Journal of Biological Chemistry. 2001 Dec 21;276(51):48341-9.

[117] De Freitas Caires N, Legendre B, Parmentier E, Scherpereel A, Tsicopoulos A, Mathieu D, et al. Identification of a 14 kDa endocan fragment generated by cathepsin G, a novel circulating biomarker in patients with sepsis. Journal of Pharmaceutical and Biomedical Analysis. 2013 May 5;78-79:45-51.

[118] Kao SJ, Chuang CY, Tang CH, Lin CH, Bien MY, Yu MC, et al. Plasma endothelial cell-specific molecule-1 (ESM-1) in management of community-acquired pneumonia. Clinical Chemistry and Laboratory Medicine. 2014 Mar;52(3):445-51.

[119] Mihajlovic DM, Lendak DF, Brkic SV, Draskovic BG, Mitic GP, Novakov Mikic AS, et al. Endocan is useful biomarker of survival and severity in sepsis. Microvascular Research. 2014 May;93:92-7.

[120] Mikkelsen ME, Shah CV, Scherpereel A, Lanken PN, Lassalle P, Bellamy SL, et al. Lower serum endocan levels are associated with the development of acute lung injury after major trauma. Journal of Critical Care. 2012 Oct;27(5):522 e11-7.

[121] Palud A, Parmentier-Decrucq E, Pastre J, De Freitas Caires N, Lassalle P, Mathieu D. Evaluation of endothelial biomarkers as predictors of organ failures in septic shock patients. Cytokine. 2015 Jun;73(2):213-8.

[122] Pauly D, Hamed S, Behnes M, Lepiorz D, Lang S, Akin I, et al. Endothelial cell-specific molecule-1/endocan: Diagnostic and prognostic value in patients suffering from severe sepsis and septic shock. Journal of Critical Care. 2016 Feb;31(1):68-75.

[123] Roldan AL, Cubellis MV, Masucci MT, Behrendt N, Lund LR, Dano K, et al. Cloning and expression of the receptor for human urokinase plasminogen activator, a central molecule in cell surface, plasmin dependent proteolysis. The EMBO Journal. 1990 Feb;9(2):467-74.

[124] Donadello K, Scolletta S, Taccone FS, Covajes C, Santonocito C, Cortes DO, et al. Soluble urokinase-type plasminogen activator receptor as a prognostic biomarker in critically ill patients. Journal of Critical Care. 2014 Feb;29(1):144-9.

[125] Hoenigl M, Raggam RB, Wagner J, Valentin T, Leitner E, Seeber K, et al. Diagnostic accuracy of soluble urokinase plasminogen activator receptor (suPAR) for prediction of bacteremia in patients with systemic inflammatory response syndrome. Clinical Biochemistry. 2013 Feb;46(3):225-9.

[126] Koch A, Voigt S, Kruschinski C, Sanson E, Duckers H, Horn A, et al. Circulating soluble urokinase plasminogen activator receptor is stably elevated during the first week of treatment in the intensive care unit and predicts mortality in critically ill patients. Critical Care. 2011;15(1):R63.

[127] Suberviola B, Castellanos-Ortega A, Ruiz Ruiz A, Lopez-Hoyos M, Santibanez M. Hospital mortality prognostication in sepsis using the new biomarkers suPAR and proADM in a single determination on ICU admission. Intensive Care Medicine. 2013 Nov;39(11):1945-52.

[128] Backes Y, van der Sluijs KF, Mackie DP, Tacke F, Koch A, Tenhunen JJ, et al. Usefulness of suPAR as a biological marker in patients with systemic inflammation or infection: A systematic review. Intensive Care Medicine. 2012 Sep;38(9):1418-28.

[129] Donadello K, Scolletta S, Covajes C, Vincent JL. suPAR as a prognostic biomarker in sepsis. BMC Medicine. 2012 Jan 05;10:2.

[130] Eugen-Olsen J, Giamarellos-Bourboulis EJ. suPAR: The unspecific marker for disease presence, severity and prognosis. International Journal of Antimicrobial Agents. 2015 Dec;46(Suppl. 1):S33-4.

[131] Huttunen R, Syrjanen J, Vuento R, Hurme M, Huhtala H, Laine J, et al. Plasma level of soluble urokinase-type plasminogen activator receptor as a predictor of disease severity and case fatality in patients with bacteraemia: A prospective cohort study. Journal of Internal Medicine. 2011 Jul;270(1):32-40.

[132] Molkanen T, Ruotsalainen E, Thorball CW, Jarvinen A. Elevated soluble urokinase plasminogen activator receptor (suPAR) predicts mortality in Staphylococcus aureus bacteremia. European Journal of Clinical Microbiology and Infectious Diseases. 2011 Nov;30(11):1417-24.

[133] Wittenhagen P, Kronborg G, Weis N, Nielsen H, Obel N, Pedersen SS, et al. The plasma level of soluble urokinase receptor is elevated in patients with *Streptococcus pneumoniae* bacteraemia and predicts mortality. Clinical Microbiology and Infection. 2004 May;10(5):409-15.

[134] Brenner T, Uhle F, Fleming T, Wieland M, Schmoch T, Schmitt F, et al. Soluble TREM-1 as a diagnostic and prognostic biomarker in patients with septic shock: An observational clinical study. Biomarkers. 2017 Feb; 22(1):63-69.

[135] Charles PE, Noel R, Massin F, Guy J, Bollaert PE, Quenot JP, et al. Significance of soluble triggering receptor expressed on myeloid cells-1 elevation in patients admitted to the intensive care unit with sepsis. BMC Infectious Diseases. 2016 Oct 12;16(1):559.

[136] Li Z, Zhang E, Hu Y, Liu Y, Chen B. High serum sTREM-1 correlates with myocardial dysfunction and predicts prognosis in septic patients. The American Journal of the Medical Sciences. 2016 Jun;351(6):555-62.

[137] Su L, Feng L, Song Q, Kang H, Zhang X, Liang Z, et al. Diagnostic value of dynamics serum sCD163, sTREM-1, PCT, and CRP in differentiating sepsis, severity assessment, and prognostic prediction. Mediators of Inflammation. 2013;2013:969875.

[138] Arizaga-Ballesteros V, Alcorta-Garcia MR, Lazaro-Martinez LC, Amezquita-Gomez JM, Alanis-Cajero JM, Villela L, et al. Can sTREM-1 predict septic shock & death in late-onset neonatal sepsis? A pilot study. International Journal of Infectious Diseases. 2015 Jan;30:27-32.

[139] Adly AA, Ismail EA, Andrawes NG, El-Saadany MA. Circulating soluble triggering receptor expressed on myeloid cells-1 (sTREM-1) as diagnostic and prognostic marker in neonatal sepsis. Cytokine. 2014 Feb;65(2):184-91.

[140] Wu Y, Wang F, Fan X, Bao R, Bo L, Li J, et al. Accuracy of plasma sTREM-1 for sepsis diagnosis in systemic inflammatory patients: A systematic review and meta-analysis. Critical Care. 2012 Nov 29;16(6):R229.

[141] Velasquez S, Matute JD, Gamez LY, Enriquez LE, Gomez ID, Toro F, et al. Characterization of nCD64 expression in neutrophils and levels of s-TREM-1 and HMGB-1 in patients with suspected infection admitted in an emergency department. Biomedica: Revista del Instituto Nacional de Salud. 2013 Oct-Dec;33(4):643-52.

[142] Su L, Liu D, Chai W, Liu D, Long Y. Role of sTREM-1 in predicting mortality of infection: A systematic review and meta-analysis. BMJ Open. 2016 May 13;6(5):e010314.

[143] Jiyong J, Tiancha H, Wei C, Huahao S. Diagnostic value of the soluble triggering receptor expressed on myeloid cells-1 in bacterial infection: A meta-analysis. Intensive Care Medicine. 2009 Apr;35(4):587-95.

[144] Orfanos SE, Maniatis NA, Kotanidou A. The effects of Activated Protein C on the Septic Syndrome. In: Vincent J-L, editor. Yearbook of Intensive Care and Emergency Medicine. Berlin, Heidelberg, New York: Springer-Verlag; 2008. pp. 721-9.

[145] Stearns-Kurosawa DJ, Kurosawa S, Mollica JS, Ferrell GL, Esmon CT. The endothelial cell protein C receptor augments protein C activation by the thrombin-thrombomodulin complex. Proceedings of the National Academy of Sciences of the United States of America. 1996 Sep 17;93(19):10212-6.

[146] Kurosawa S, Stearns-Kurosawa DJ, Carson CW, D'Angelo A, Della Valle P, Esmon CT. Plasma levels of endothelial cell protein C receptor are elevated in patients with sepsis and systemic lupus erythematosus: Lack of correlation with thrombomodulin suggests involvement of different pathological processes. Blood. 1998 Jan 15;91(2):725-7.

[147] Liaw PC, Esmon CT, Kahnamoui K, Schmidt S, Kahnamoui S, Ferrell G, et al. Patients with severe sepsis vary markedly in their ability to generate activated protein C. Blood. 2004 Dec 15;104(13):3958-64.

[148] Faust SN, Levin M, Harrison OB, Goldin RD, Lockhart MS, Kondaveeti S, et al. Dysfunction of endothelial protein C activation in severe meningococcal sepsis. The New England Journal of Medicine. 2001 Aug 9;345(6):408-16.

[149] Borgel D, Bornstain C, Reitsma PH, Lerolle N, Gandrille S, Dali-Ali F, et al. A comparative study of the protein C pathway in septic and nonseptic patients with organ failure. The American Journal of Respiratory and Critical Care Medicine. 2007 Nov 1; 176(9):878-85.

[150] Kager LM, Schouten M, Wiersinga WJ, de Boer JD, Lattenist LC, Roelofs JJ, et al. Overexpression of the Endothelial Protein C Receptor Is Detrimental during Pneumonia-Derived Gram-negative Sepsis (Melioidosis). PLoS Neglected Tropical Diseases. 2013 Jul;7(7):e2306.

[151] Guitton C, Gerard N, Sebille V, Bretonniere C, Zambon O, Villers D, et al. Early rise in circulating endothelial protein C receptor correlates with poor outcome in severe sepsis. Intensive Care Medicine. 2011 Jun;37(6):950-6.

[152] Vassiliou AG, Kotanidou A, Mastora Z, Maniatis NA, Albani P, Jahaj E, et al. Elevated soluble endothelial protein C receptor levels at ICU admission are associated with sepsis development. Minerva Anestesiologica. 2015 Feb;81(2):125-34.

[153] Ulla M, Pizzolato E, Lucchiari M, Loiacono M, Soardo F, Forno D, et al. Diagnostic and prognostic value of presepsin in the management of sepsis in the emergency department: A multicenter prospective study. Critical Care. 2013 Jul 30;17(4):R168.

[154] Okamura Y. Usefulness of presepsin measurement: A new biomarker for sepsis. Rinsho Byori. 2015 Jan;63(1):62-71.

[155] Endo S, Suzuki Y, Takahashi G, Shozushima T, Ishikura H, Murai A, et al. Usefulness of presepsin in the diagnosis of sepsis in a multicenter prospective study. Journal of Infection and Chemotherapy. 2012 Dec;18(6):891-7.

[156] Behnes M, Bertsch T, Lepiorz D, Lang S, Trinkmann F, Brueckmann M, et al. Diagnostic and prognostic utility of soluble CD 14 subtype (presepsin) for severe sepsis and septic shock during the first week of intensive care treatment. Critical Care. 2014 Sep 05;18(5):507.

[157] Masson S, Caironi P, Spanuth E, Thomae R, Panigada M, Sangiorgi G, et al. Presepsin (soluble CD14 subtype) and procalcitonin levels for mortality prediction in sepsis: Data from the Albumin Italian Outcome Sepsis trial. Critical Care. 2014 Jan 07;18(1):R6.

[158] Zhang J, Hu ZD, Song J, Shao J. Diagnostic value of presepsin for sepsis: A systematic review and meta-analysis. Medicine. 2015 Nov;94(47):e2158.

[159] Zheng Z, Jiang L, Ye L, Gao Y, Tang L, Zhang M. The accuracy of presepsin for the diagnosis of sepsis from SIRS: A systematic review and meta-analysis. Annals of Intensive Care. 2015 Dec;5(1):48.

[160] Wu J, Hu L, Zhang G, Wu F, He T. Accuracy of Presepsin in Sepsis Diagnosis: A systematic review and meta-analysis. PLoS One. 2015;10(7):e0133057.

[161] Ali FT, Ali MA, Elnakeeb MM, Bendary HN. Presepsin is an early monitoring biomarker for predicting clinical outcome in patients with sepsis. Clinica Chimica Acta. 2016 Sep 01;460:93-101.

[162] Klouche K, Cristol JP, Devin J, Gilles V, Kuster N, Larcher R, et al. Diagnostic and prognostic value of soluble CD14 subtype (Presepsin) for sepsis and community-acquired pneumonia in ICU patients. Annals of Intensive Care. 2016 Dec;6(1):59.

[163] Leli C, Ferranti M, Marrano U, Al Dhahab ZS, Bozza S, Cenci E, et al. Diagnostic accuracy of presepsin (sCD14-ST) and procalcitonin for prediction of bacteraemia and bacterial DNAaemia in patients with suspected sepsis. Journal of Medical Microbiology. 2016 Aug;65(8):713-9.

[164] Franekova J, Secnik P, Jr., Lavrikova P, Kubicek Z, Hoskova L, Kieslichova E, et al. Serial measurement of presepsin, procalcitonin, and C-reactive protein in the early postoperative period and the response to antithymocyte globulin administration after heart transplantation. Clinical Transplantation. 2017 Jan;31(1): e12870.

[165] de Guadiana Romualdo LG, Torrella PE, Acebes SR, Oton MD, Sanchez RJ, Holgado AH, et al. Diagnostic accuracy of presepsin (sCD14-ST) as a biomarker of infection and sepsis in the emergency department. Clinica Chimica Acta. 2017 Jan;464:6-11.

[166] Montaldo P, Rosso R, Santantonio A, Chello G, Giliberti P. Presepsin for the detection of early-onset sepsis in preterm newborns. Pediatric Research. 2017 Feb;81(2):329-334.

[167] Ozdemir AA, Elgormus Y. Diagnostic Value of Presepsin in Detection of Early-Onset Neonatal Sepsis. The American Journal of Perinatology. 2016 Nov 08. DOI: 10.1055/s-0036-1593851.

[168] Pugni L, Pietrasanta C, Milani S, Vener C, Ronchi A, Falbo M, et al. Presepsin (Soluble CD14 Subtype): Reference ranges of a new sepsis marker in term and preterm neonates. PLoS One. 2015;10(12):e0146020.

[169] Arnold RC, Shapiro NI, Jones AE, Schorr C, Pope J, Casner E, et al. Multicenter study of early lactate clearance as a determinant of survival in patients with presumed sepsis. Shock. 2009 Jul;32(1):35-9.

[170] Nguyen HB, Rivers EP, Knoblich BP, Jacobsen G, Muzzin A, Ressler JA, et al. Early lactate clearance is associated with improved outcome in severe sepsis and septic shock. Critical Care Medicine. 2004 Aug;32(8):1637-42.

[171] Singer AJ, Taylor M, Domingo A, Ghazipura S, Khorasonchi A, Thode HC, Jr., et al. Diagnostic characteristics of a clinical screening tool in combination with measuring bedside lactate level in emergency department patients with suspected sepsis. Academic Emergency Medicine. 2014 Aug;21(8):853-7.

[172] Bakker J, Gris P, Coffernils M, Kahn RJ, Vincent JL. Serial blood lactate levels can predict the development of multiple organ failure following septic shock. The American Journal of Surgery. 1996 Feb;171(2):221-6.

[173] Mikkelsen ME, Miltiades AN, Gaieski DF, Goyal M, Fuchs BD, Shah CV, et al. Serum lactate is associated with mortality in severe sepsis independent of organ failure and shock. Critical Care Medicine. 2009 May;37(5):1670-7.

[174] Shapiro NI, Howell MD, Talmor D, Nathanson LA, Lisbon A, Wolfe RE, et al. Serum lactate as a predictor of mortality in emergency department patients with infection. Annals of Emergency Medicine. 2005 May;45(5):524-8.

[175] Trzeciak S, Dellinger RP, Chansky ME, Arnold RC, Schorr C, Milcarek B, et al. Serum lactate as a predictor of mortality in patients with infection. Intensive Care Medicine. 2007 Jun;33(6):970-7.

[176] Singer AJ, Taylor M, LeBlanc D, Williams J, Thode HC, Jr. ED bedside point-of-care lactate in patients with suspected sepsis is associated with reduced time to iv fluids and mortality. The American Journal of Emergency Medicine. 2014 Sep;32(9):1120-4.

[177] Levraut J, Ciebiera JP, Chave S, Rabary O, Jambou P, Carles M, et al. Mild hyperlactatemia in stable septic patients is due to impaired lactate clearance rather than overproduction. The American Journal of Respiratory and Critical Care Medicine. 1998 Apr;157(4 Pt 1):1021-6.

[178] Revelly JP, Tappy L, Martinez A, Bollmann M, Cayeux MC, Berger MM, et al. Lactate and glucose metabolism in severe sepsis and cardiogenic shock. Critical Care Medicine. 2005 Oct;33(10):2235-40.

[179] Scott HF, Donoghue AJ, Gaieski DF, Marchese RF, Mistry RD. The utility of early lactate testing in undifferentiated pediatric systemic inflammatory response syndrome. Academic Emergency Medicine. 2012 Nov;19(11):1276-80.

[180] Vassiliou AG, Mastora Z, Jahaj E, Koutsoukou A, Orfanos SE, Kotanidou A. Does serum lactate combined with soluble endothelial selectins at ICU admission predict sepsis development? In Vivo. 2015 Mar–Apr;29(2):305-8.

[181] Kofoed K, Andersen O, Kronborg G, Tvede M, Petersen J, Eugen-Olsen J, et al. Use of plasma C-reactive protein, procalcitonin, neutrophils, macrophage migration inhibitory factor, soluble urokinase-type plasminogen activator receptor, and soluble triggering receptor expressed on myeloid cells-1 in combination to diagnose infections: A prospective study. Critical Care. 2007;11(2):R38.

[182] Shapiro NI, Trzeciak S, Hollander JE, Birkhahn R, Otero R, Osborn TM, et al. A prospective, multicenter derivation of a biomarker panel to assess risk of organ dysfunction, shock, and death in emergency department patients with suspected sepsis. Critical Care Medicine. 2009 Jan;37(1):96-104.

[183] Andaluz-Ojeda D, Bobillo F, Iglesias V, Almansa R, Rico L, Gandía F, et al. A combined score of pro- and anti-inflammatory interleukins improves mortality prediction in severe sepsis. Cytokine. 2012;57:332-6.

[184] Gogos CA, Drosou E, Bassaris HP, Skoutelis A. Pro- versus anti-inflammatory cytokine profile in patients with severe sepsis: A marker for prognosis and future therapeutic options. Journal of Infectious Diseases. 2000 Jan;181(1):176-80. PubMed PMID: 10608764. Epub 1999/12/23. Eng.

[185] Sutherland AM, Walley KR. Bench-to-bedside review: Association of genetic variation with sepsis. Critical Care. 2009;13(2):210.

[186] Villar J, Maca-Meyer N, Perez-Mendez L, Flores C. Bench-to-bedside review: Underst anding genetic predisposition to sepsis. Critical Care. 2004 Jun;8(3):180-9.

[187] Takeda K, Akira S. Toll-like receptors in innate immunity. International Immunology. 2005 Jan;17(1):1-14. PubMed PMID: 15585605. Epub 2004/12/09. Eng.

[188] Poltorak A, He X, Smirnova I, Liu MY, Van Huffel C, Du X, et al. Defective LPS signaling in C3H/HeJ and C57BL/10ScCr mice: Mutations in Tlr4 gene. Science. 1998 Dec 11;282(5396):2085-8.

[189] Hoshino K, Takeuchi O, Kawai T, Sanjo H, Ogawa T, Takeda Y, et al. Pillars article: Cutting edge: Toll-like receptor 4 (TLR4)-deficient mice are hyporesponsive to lipopolysaccharide: Evidence for TLR4 as the Lps gene product. Journal of Immunology. 1999;162:3749-52. Journal of Immunology. 2016 Oct 1;197(7):2563-6.

[190] Feterowski C, Emmanuilidis K, Miethke T, Gerauer K, Rump M, Ulm K, et al. Effects of functional Toll-like receptor-4 mutations on the immune response to human and experimental sepsis. Immunology. 2003 Jul;109(3):426-31.

[191] Smirnova I, Mann N, Dols A, Derkx HH, Hibberd ML, Levin M, et al. Assay of locus-specific genetic load implicates rare Toll-like receptor 4 mutations in meningococcal susceptibility. Proceedings of the National Academy of Sciences of the United States of America. 2003 May 13;100(10):6075-80.

[192] Lorenz E, Mira JP, Frees KL, Schwartz DA. Relevance of mutations in the TLR4 receptor in patients with gram-negative septic shock. Archives of Internal Medicine. 2002 May 13;162(9):1028-32.

[193] Kiechl S, Lorenz E, Reindl M, Wiedermann CJ, Oberhollenzer F, Bonora E, et al. Toll-like receptor 4 polymorphisms and atherogenesis. The New England Journal of Medicine. 2002 Jul 18;347(3):185-92.

[194] Yousef AA, Suliman GA, Mabrouk MM. The value of admission serum IL-8 monitoring and the correlation with IL-8 (−251A/T) polymorphism in critically ill patients. ISRN Inflammation. 2014 Mar;6:494985.

[195] Belopolskaya OB, Smelaya TV, Moroz VV, Golubev AM, Salnikova LE. Clinical associations of host genetic variations in the genes of cytokines in critically ill patients. Clinical & Experimental Immunology. 2015 Jun;180(3):531-41.

[196] Abu-Maziad A, Schaa K, Bell EF, Dagle JM, Cooper M, Marazita ML, et al. Role of polymorphic variants as genetic modulators of infection in neonatal sepsis. Pediatric Research. 2010 Oct;68(4):323-9.

[197] Esposito S, Zampiero A, Pugni L, Tabano S, Pelucchi C, Ghirardi B, et al. Genetic polymorphisms and sepsis in premature neonates. PLoS One. 2014;9(7):e101248.

[198] Hu D, Wang H, Huang X, Jiang Y, Qin Y, Xiong B, et al. Investigation of association between IL-8 serum levels and IL8 polymorphisms in Chinese patients with sepsis. Gene. 2016 Dec 5;594(1):165-70.

[199] Mira JP, Cariou A, Grall F, Delclaux C, Losser MR, Heshmati F, et al. Association of TNF-2, a TNF-alpha promoter polymorphism, with septic shock susceptibility and mortality: A multicenter study. The Journal of the American Medical Association. 1999 Aug 11;282(6):561-8.

[200] Stuber F, Petersen M, Bokelmann F, Schade U. A genomic polymorphism within the tumor necrosis factor locus influences plasma tumor necrosis factor-alpha concentrations and outcome of patients with severe sepsis. Critical Care Medicine. 1996 Mar;24(3):381-4.

[201] Teuffel O, Ethier MC, Beyene J, Sung L. Association between tumor necrosis factor-alpha promoter −308 A/G polymorphism and susceptibility to sepsis and sepsis mortality: A systematic review and meta-analysis. Critical Care Medicine. 2010 Jan;38(1):276-82.

[202] Gordon AC, Lagan AL, Aganna E, Cheung L, Peters CJ, McDermott MF, et al. TNF and TNF-R polymorphisms in severe sepsis and septic shock: A prospective multicentre study. Genes and Immunity. 2004 Dec;5(8):631-40.

[203] Carvalho JK, Moore DB, Luz RA, Xavier-Elsas PP, Gaspar-Elsas MI. Prediction of sepsis-related outcomes in neonates through systematic genotyping of polymorphisms in genes for innate immunity and inflammation: A narrative review and critical perspective. Sao Paulo Medical Journal = Revista paulista de medicina. 2013;131(5):338-50.

[204] Fishman D, Faulds G, Jeffery R, Mohamed-Ali V, Yudkin JS, Humphries S, et al. The effect of novel polymorphisms in the interleukin-6 (IL-6) gene on IL-6 transcription and plasma IL-6 levels, and an association with systemic-onset juvenile chronic arthritis. Journal of Clinical Investigation. 1998 Oct 1;102(7):1369-76.

[205] Gaudino M, Andreotti F, Zamparelli R, Di Castelnuovo A, Nasso G, Burzotta F, et al. The -174G/C interleukin-6 polymorphism influences postoperative interleukin-6 levels and postoperative atrial fibrillation. Is atrial fibrillation an inflammatory complication? Circulation. 2003 Sep 9;108(Suppl. 1):II195-9.

[206] Roth-Isigkeit A, Hasselbach L, Ocklitz E, Bruckner S, Ros A, Gehring H, et al. Inter-individual differences in cytokine release in patients undergoing cardiac surgery with cardiopulmonary bypass. Clinical & Experimental Immunology. 2001 Jul;125(1):80-8.

[207] Schluter B, Raufhake C, Erren M, Schotte H, Kipp F, Rust S, et al. Effect of the interleukin-6 promoter polymorphism (−174 G/C) on the incidence and outcome of sepsis. Critical Care Medicine. 2002 Jan;30(1):32-7.

[208] Sutherland AM, Walley KR, Manocha S, Russell JA. The association of interleukin 6 haplotype clades with mortality in critically ill adults. Archives of Internal Medicine. 2005 Jan 10;165(1):75-82.

[209] Chauhan M, McGuire W. Interleukin-6 (−174C) polymorphism and the risk of sepsis in very low birth weight infants: Meta-analysis. Archives of Disease in Childhood Fetal and Neonatal Edition. 2008 Nov;93(6):F427-9.

[210] John Baier R, Loggins J, Yanamandra K. Angiotensin converting enzyme insertion/deletion polymorphism does not alter sepsis outcome in ventilated very low birth weight infants. Journal of Perinatology. 2005 Mar;25(3):205-9.

[211] Spiegler J, Gilhaus A, Konig IR, Kattner E, Vochem M, Kuster H, et al. Polymorphisms in the Renin-Angiotensin system and outcome of very-low-birthweight infants. Neonatology. 2010;97(1):10-4.

[212] Cogulu O, Onay H, Uzunkaya D, Gunduz C, Pehlivan S, Vardar F, et al. Role of angiotensin-converting enzyme gene polymorphisms in children with sepsis and septic shock. Pediatrics International. 2008 Aug;50(4):477-80.

[213] Yang H, Wang Y, Liu L, Hu Q. Increased susceptibility of sepsis associated with CD143 deletion/insertion polymorphism in Caucasians: A meta analysis. International Journal of Clinical and Experimental Pathology. 2014;7(10):6551-8.

[214] Hou X, Zhang P, Nie W, Tang S, Wang J, Zhang Q, et al. Association between angiotensin-converting enzyme I/D polymorphism and sepsis: A meta-analysis. Journal of the Renin-Angiotensin-Aldosterone System. 2015 Jun;16(2):415-21.

[215] Tsantes A, Tsangaris I, Kopterides P, Nikolopoulos G, Kalamara E, Antonakos G, et al. Angiotensin converting enzyme (ACE) insertion/deletion (I/D) polymorphism and circulating ACE levels are not associated with outcome in critically ill septic patients. Clinical Chemistry and Laboratory Medicine. 2011 Oct 21;50(2):293-9.

[216] Villar J, Flores C, Perez-Mendez L, Maca-Meyer N, Espinosa E, Blanco J, et al. Angiotensin-converting enzyme insertion/deletion polymorphism is not associated with susceptibility and outcome in sepsis and acute respiratory distress syndrome. Intensive Care Medicine. 2008 Mar;34(3):488-95.

[217] Cardinal-Fernandez P, Ferruelo A, El-Assar M, Santiago C, Gomez-Gallego F, Martin-Pellicer A, et al. Genetic predisposition to acute respiratory distress syndrome in patients with severe sepsis. Shock. 2013 Mar;39(3):255-60.

[218] Sipahi T, Pocan H, Akar N. Effect of various genetic polymorphisms on the incidence and outcome of severe sepsis. Clinical and Applied Thrombosis/Hemostasis. 2006 Jan;12(1):47-54.

[219] Vassiliou AG, Maniatis NA, Kotanidou A, Kallergi M, Karystinaki FS, Letsiou E, et al. Endothelial protein C receptor polymorphisms and risk of severe sepsis in critically ill patients. Intensive Care Medicine. 2013 Oct;39(10):1752-9.

Chapter 7

In Vivo Imaging of Septic Encephalopathy

Yukio Imamura, Yuki Murakami, Naoya Matsumoto,
Hisatake Matsumoto, Satoko Mitani,
Kentaro Shimizu, Hiroshi Ogura,
Takeshi Shimazu and Takashi Jin

Additional information is available at the end of the chapter

http://dx.doi.org/10.5772/67983

Abstract

Septic encephalopathy is a devastating symptom of severe sepsis. Many studies have been performed to uncover the pathophysiological mechanisms of septic encephalopathy; however, novel technical approaches are still required to overcome this complex symptom. Because patients are suffering from severe cognitive impairment, coma, or delirium, which burden not only patients but also caregivers, overcoming septic encephalopathy is still a major social problem worldwide, especially in the intensive care. Septic encephalopathy seems to be caused by cytokine invasion and/or oxidative stress into the brain, and this pathological state leads to imbalance of neurotransmitters. In addition to this pathophysiology, septic encephalopathy causes complicated symptoms (e.g., ischemic stroke, edema, and aberrant sensory function). For these pathophysiological mechanisms, electrophysiology using animal models, positron emission tomography (PET), computed tomography, and magnetic resonance imaging for septic patients has provided important clues. However, the research for septic encephalopathy is currently confronted with the difficulty of complex symptoms. To overcome this situation, in this chapter, we introduce our novel methods for in vivo imaging of septic encephalopathy using near infrared (NIR) nanoparticles, quantum dots. In addition to our recent progress, we propose a strategy for the future approach to in vivo imaging of septic encephalopathy.

Keywords: septic encephalopathy, molecular mechanism, in vivo imaging, quantum dots, disseminated intravascular coagulation

1. Introduction

Although the pathophysiological mechanism of septic encephalopathy (SE) still includes some mystery, recent progress of challenging research using animal models of sepsis has

INTECH
open science | open minds

© 2017 The Author(s). Licensee InTech. This chapter is distributed under the terms of the Creative Commons Attribution License (http://creativecommons.org/licenses/by/3.0), which permits unrestricted use, distribution, and reproduction in any medium, provided the original work is properly cited.

gradually uncovered the molecular pathogenesis of SE. For instance, recent pathophysiological findings for SE include synaptic deficiency by interleukin-1 beta [1] and acetylcholine [2] and brain ischemia or edema with disseminated intravascular coagulation (DIC) [3]. These phenomena are dynamically altered in a time-dependent manner based on the content of symptoms. Functional magnetic resonance imaging (fMRI) for patients of SE can describe the status of symptoms; however, it is difficult to track these time-dependent changes in the septic brain because of the low time resolution of its measurement. To overcome this technical difficulty, we are working to develop noninvasive near infrared (NIR) imaging as a novel method to analyze the pathological state of SE.

In this chapter, we introduce current understanding of pathophysiology, the imaging technology, and the application of novel imaging technology to visualize the pathophysiological mechanism of SE. The contents are described as follows: (1) etiology of SE, (2) molecular mechanisms of pathogenesis, (3) NIR in vivo imaging, and (4) application to SE. In particular, we focus on DIC and our approach firstly demonstrates the novel application of NIR in vivo imaging to DIC. We expect that this review will be helpful to readers such as basic biomedical students, and scientists who are interested in the future preclinical and clinical application to SE.

2. Septic encephalopathy (SE)

Septic encephalopathy (SE) is a symptom with brain dysfunction caused by sepsis. Up to 70% of severe septic patients encountered developed SE [4]. Patients with SE are often suffering from various neurological symptoms. Many research reports and reviews have discussed cognitive impairment [5, 6], delirium [7], coma [8–11], and recently seizure and aberrant sensory function [12–16]. In addition, complication symptoms such as ischemic stroke, edema, etc. occurred [17–19]. However, not all of pathophysiological mechanisms for SE have been clarified in Ref. [20], and a better understanding of SE is still an important social problem worldwide [21].

2.1. Etiology

The SE is often found in acute liver failure and cirrhosis patients and triggered by the various chemical mediators followed by systemic inflammatory response syndromes, whole-body inflammation [22–24]. SE is different from the brain "encephalitis" which occurs due to pathogens (e.g., bacteria, virus, etc.) direct invasion into the brain. Rather than the direct invasion, SE is caused indirectly by excessive inflammatory response (e.g., cytokine storm). Thus, SE is a symptom. Clinical studies for SE reported that patients with SE often suffered from hypotension [25], imbalance of amino acids in plasma [26], and neuronal injury with edema [27, 28]. Several lines of evidences suggest that a rodent model of SE showed aberrant behavior: altered sensory function [29, 30], increased anxiety [31, 32], and cognitive impairment [33]. These results are similar to the symptoms of brain dysfunction in SE patients [34]. Thus, neurological impairment leads to various symptoms in SE.

3. Molecular mechanisms

3.1. Pathogenesis

To understand the molecular mechanisms, pathophysiological factors (e.g., imbalance of chemical substances, cellular environment, and molecules) are discussed. Overall pathogenesis for SE is summarized in **Figure 1**. When SE is occurred, various chemical substances (e.g., neurotransmitter, modulator, etc.) were involved as reviewed elsewhere in Refs. [35, 36]. These chemical substances were mainly important for maintaining homeostasis in the normal condition. After the SE occurred, the imbalanced rate of substances (e.g., amino acids) [37–41] abrogated brain metabolic function (e.g., tryptophan metabolism) [42–44], microglial activation in the brain followed by detachment of pericyte from microvascular basal lamina [45, 46].

Normally, the brain is protected with a barrier called blood brain barrier (BBB). The barrier consists of brain endothelial cells, and these cells are tightly attached with tight junction. The barrier is selectively permeable to transport of amino acid, gas, and lipid-soluble chemicals which are important for neuronal function. Therefore, the inflammatory molecules cannot affect brain function in the normal condition because the brain is protected with blood brain barrier, and foreign substances are impeded by this barrier.

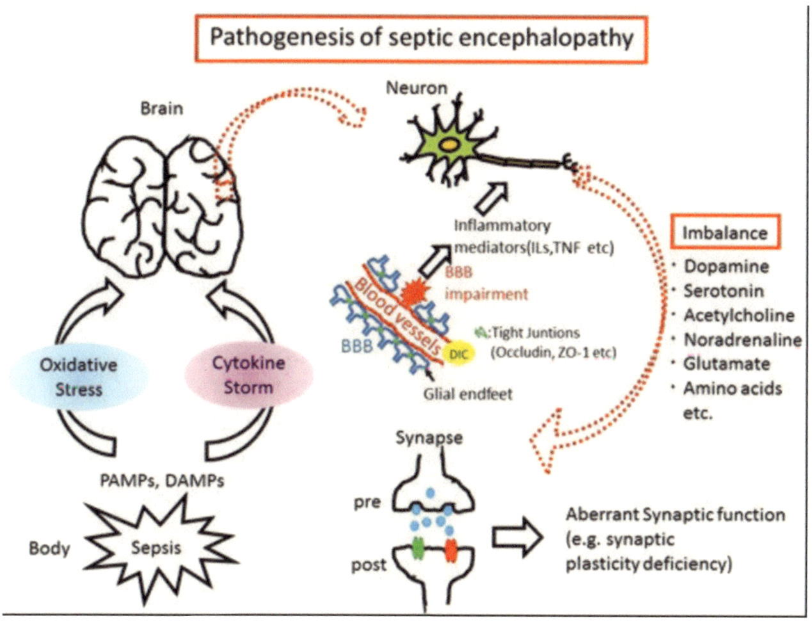

Figure 1. Overview of pathogenesis for septic encephalopathy (SE). Severe sepsis often results in septic encephalopathy, mainly followed by oxidative stress and cytokine storm. Accompanying BBB impairment and DIC, invaded inflammatory mediators cause aberrant neuronal function. PAMPs: pathogen-associated molecular pattern; DAMPs: damage-associated molecular patterns; BBB: blood brain barrier; IL: interleukin; TNF: tumor necrosis factor.

In the septic condition, occurrence of systemic inflammatory response syndromes is followed by sepsis, the syndromes lead to destruction of this blood brain barrier [47, 48], and harmful chemical substances disrupt normal brain function. Then, the chemical substances cause the aberrant neuronal transmission and plasticity [1, 30]. The components of tight junctions are claudin, occludin, zona occludin, etc. [49]. This tight junction serves as if an adhesive of cells and underpins the blood brain barriers. Using a mouse model of sepsis, we clearly demonstrated that the occludin protein was destroyed 20 h after induction of sepsis and led to a permeabilization of cytokine [1, 30]. Other groups reported that tumor necrosis factor (TNF)-alpha and calcium-binding proteins were increased in the SE [50].

3.2. Blood brain barrier (BBB) impairment

Why was the tight junction disrupted? Overall mechanisms are still unclear, a hypothesis is, however, addressed. Neuroinflammation (e.g., microglia/macrophage activation, nitrogen oxide gas production) resulted in the mitochondria dysfunction with reactive oxygen synthesis (ROS) [51–55] and dysfunction of cerebrovascular endothelial cells [56]. The process is impeded by ROS inhibitors [57] or mitochondria-targeted peptides [55].

Another hypothesis is as follows. Septic patients sometimes showed a rapid vasoconstriction of blood vessels, and this mechanical alteration may cause the damage to the microvasculature structure [58, 59]. Endothelin and its receptor which constrict blood vessels might be involved in that process [60, 61]. Phosphoinositide 3-kinase cascade activated microglial cell and matrix metalloproteinase (i.e., marker of inflammation) and aggravated BBB impairment [62]. Consequently, the BBB disruption finally leads to the invasion of inflammatory mediators into the brain of SE [63].

3.3. Effect of cytokine storm on brain function

In any case, the dysfunction of blood brain barrier after sepsis increases the permeability of inflammatory molecules as described below and finally causes the brain malfunction.

For example, there are widely discussed cytokines such as interleukins (interleukin-1, -6, -10) [37, 64], tumor necrosis factor (TNF)-alpha [65, 66], complement C5a [67], and cascade [68]. Epigenetic modulation (e.g., histone acetylation) participates in the trigger of aberrant glutamate receptor subunits [29, 69] and causes memory deficit [70]. In addition, disseminated blood coagulation [71, 72] and oxidative stress [73–75] aggravated brain dysfunction of SE. MicroRNA (i.e., noncoding small RNA) involved in RNA silencing and posttranscriptional modification [76]. Besides nitric oxide (NO), lipid peroxidase, S100B protein [77], and the prion protein [78] may participate in SE.

3.4. Imbalance of synaptic transmissions on neurons

As a morphological study revealed that the neuronal spine was destabilized in a mouse model [79], neuronal environment may possibly be altered in SE. Actually, for other potent factors related to neurotransmission, norepinephrine [80], adrenergic system [81, 82], serotonergic system [83], acetylcholine [84–86], gamma-aminobutyric receptor A [87], N-methyl-D-aspartate receptor 2B [29], and brain neurovascular dysfunction [88] were involved in the pathogenesis of SE. In summary, sepsis leads to the aberrant conditions in the neuronal and/or glial environments and may result in the devastating symptoms in the pathogenesis of SE.

4. Brain activity measurements: from electrophysiology to imaging

4.1. Electrophysiology

Neurophysiological studies have uncovered the neuronal dysfunction in SE. Neurophysiologists have developed various experimental techniques to study neuronal cell activity. Neuronal activities recordings can be classified as follows: (1) single neuronal activity and (2) multiple neuronal activity. To record the single neuronal activity, there are techniques such as patch clamp recording and intracellular recording.

On the other hand, to record multiple neuronal activity, there are several established techniques. For example, there are field excitatory postsynaptic potentials (in vitro), local field potential (in vivo), and optical recording with voltage sensitive dye (in vitro and in vivo). For example, Kafa et al. reported reduced neuronal population activities in a rat model of SE [89], and Wang et al. also showed suppression of local field potentials during sensory stimulation in SE [30]. These findings are clearly similar to the clinical state of sensory dysfunction in septic patients [90]. It is useful to uncover the pathophysiological mechanism. These techniques are very powerful for studying the single neuron or several neurons in the local region of the brain. However, symptoms of SE are versatile with complicated diseases (e.g., stroke, edema, myopathy, etc.) [35, 91, 92]. Integrative analysis with multiple viewpoints is still required [93].

4.2. Brain imaging

Noninvasive measurement was sought to determine the pathological state and followed by prognosis of SE [94]. Several research reports suggest that electroencephalogram (EEG) that placed to the surface of head was useful to study brain dysfunction by various encephalitis and encephalopathy [95, 96]. In SE, for example, the EEG recordings revealed decreased amplitudes of EEG signals [97]. Using a rat model, EEG signals were attenuated [83]. In addition, child patient with coma showed 6-Hz burst firing pattern in SE [98]. Hence, EEG abnormality was found in the SE [99].

Why have these altered activity patterns due to brain dysfunction occurred? Functional magnetic resonance imaging (fMRI) has been used to capture the pathological state of brain cortex in SE [100]. Clinically, patients of SE showed cerebral infarction with multiple ischemic stroke and white matter lesions [13, 101]. Additionally, cerebral edema was reported [102]. Recently, brain atrophy within the regions including amygdala, hippocampus, basal ganglia, brainstem, thalamic, and cerebellar neurons was also shown in Ref. [103, 104]. Hence, complicated symptoms, if they represent irreversible morphological alteration, have been found with fMRI. In addition to fMRI, positron emission tomography (PET) using 18 F-FDG was applied [105]; however, the application was limited. Conversely, reversible and time-dependent altered symptoms (e.g., neuronal transmission) cannot be determined with fMRI imaging (and PET) [106]. Because fMRI takes 10–30 min or more to capture a brain image with the high spatial resolution, it only determines the stable state of the pathology for SE. To overcome this weak point, we are currently focused on the noninvasive NIR imaging.

5. Near infrared (NIR) in vivo imaging

5.1. Probes

NIR imaging is a powerful tool for noninvasive in vivo imaging. Conventionally, visible light (400–700 nm) has been used for molecular fluorescent imaging in cellular dynamics [107, 108]. However, visible light is difficult to apply to deep-tissue imaging because of the robust light absorption and scattering by intrinsic chromophores (hemoglobin, melanin, flavin, etc.) and organelles (mitochondria and cytoskeleton). Autofluorescence from tissues (heart, skin, and brain) which is excited by NIR light (700–1400 nm) is much lower than that by excited visible light [109]. In addition, NIR light permeates tissues more than visible light (400–700 nm) (**Figure 2**). Therefore, the NIR light, especially 2nd optical window (1000–1400 nm), is currently expected to be applicable to noninvasive deep tissue imaging.

To label the target tissue, fluorescent probes are necessary. Compared to the visible light probes, NIR fluorescence probes are limited. For example, single-walled carbon nanotubes (SWNTs), Ag_2S quantum dots, PbS quantum dots, and rare-earth-doped nanocomposites are developed for 2nd optical windows for in vivo imaging (reviewed in Ref. [110]). We previously

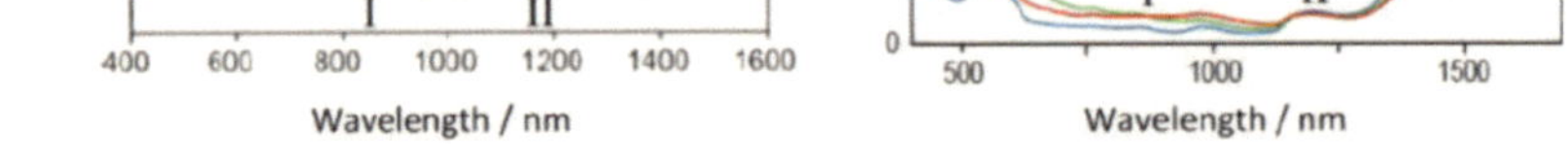

Figure 2. (a) Autofluorescence spectra of the dorsal side of a mouse body. The autofluorescence spectra were taken by excitation of 482, 670, and 785 nm. The dotted and solid arrows show the wavelength rage of 1st NIR optical window (I) and 2nd NIR optical window (II), respectively. (b) Absorption spectra of tissue slices of mouse skin, brain, and heart. Slice thickness of the skin, brain, and heart is 120, 100, and 200 μm, respectively. (Citation from Ref. [110]).

compared these fluorescence probes in the same condition and found that PbS quantum dots were much brighter than other probes (**Figure 3**).

5.2. In vivo imaging

We applied PbS quantum dots (maximum fluorescence intensity: 1100 nm) from mouse tail vein and successfully recorded blood flow in the mouse head in a noninvasive manner [71] (**Figure 4**). The head of an anesthetized mouse was fixed on a stage of a microscope, and fluorescence was recorded through skin and skull (**Figure 4a**). The fluorescent intensity was recorded with InGaAs camera which is sensitive from 900–1600 nm. Soon after injection, brain blood vessels were visible on a mouse head (**Figure 4b**, right), and the picture was entirely similar to the image of blood vessels after scalp removal (**Figure 4c**, upper) and isolated brain (**Figure 4c**, lower). These findings suggest that the NIR in vivo imaging can visualize the brain blood flow non-invasively. If we would like to apply this method to the pathophysiology of SE, what is the target?

Brain blood vessels are aggravated in SE. Previous reports addressed that, using an animal model, cerebral microcirculation was reported to be impaired [111]. Disseminated intravascular coagulation (DIC) is an important pathological state of sepsis and worsening of DIC increases multiple organ dysfunction. Anticoagulant therapy was performed, however, its effect was limited. Repetitive administration of anticoagulant drug increases the rate of side effects such as thrombocytopenia [112] and bleeding [113]. To find the pathological state of DIC, we examined whether NIR in vivo imaging detect DIC in the septic brain as described in the next section.

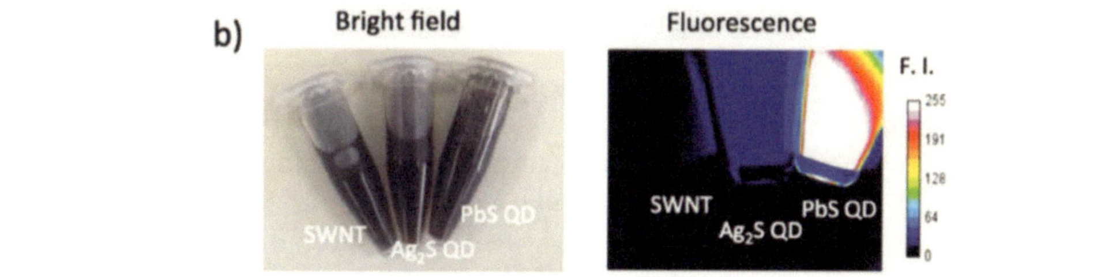

Figure 3. (a) Fluorescence spectra of nanomaterials that emit in the 2nd NIR window: SWNT, Ag_2S QD, and PbS QD. (b) Bright field and fluorescence images (>1000 nm) of SWNT, Ag_2S QD, and PbS QD. To compare the fluorescence brightness, absorbance at the excitation wavelength (720 nm) was adjusted to be the same value of 0.5 for SWNT, Ag_2S QD, and PbS QD. (Citation from Ref. [110]).

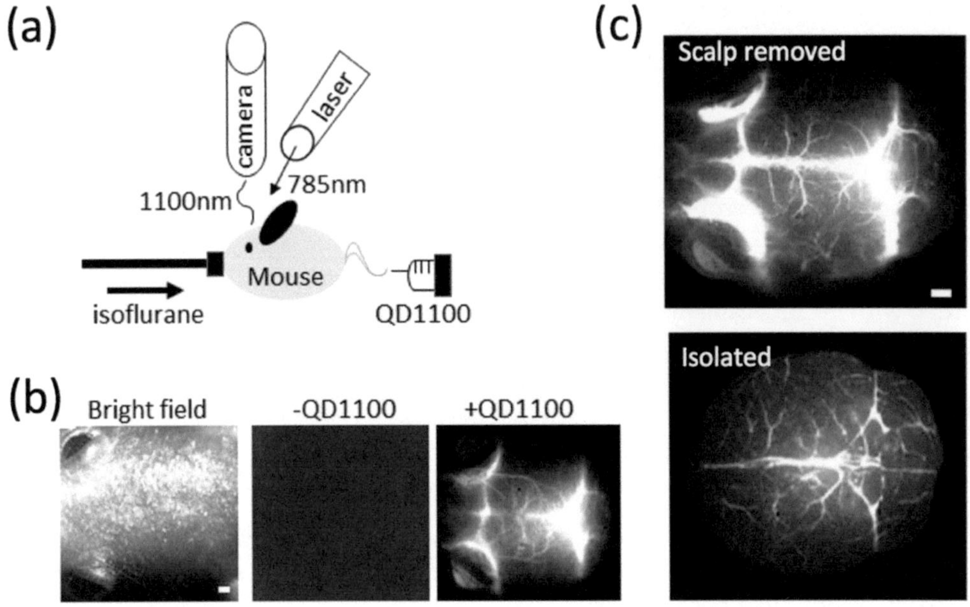

Figure 4. (a) Experimental setup for NIR fluorescence imaging of cerebral blood vessels. An anesthetized mouse was administered QD1100 in a caudal vein. An optical laser (785 nm wavelength) was used as an excitation light source, and NIR fluorescence was detected with an InGaAs camera; (b) imaging of a mouse head. Bright field image (left), NIR fluorescence image without QD administration (middle), and the NIR fluorescence image with QD administration (right). Scale bar: 1 mm; (c) NIR fluorescence images of cerebral blood vessels. Upper: fluorescence image after scalp removed, lower: fluorescence image after isolation. Scale bars: 1 mm. (Citation from Ref. [71]).

6. Application of NIR in vivo imaging to pathological analyses for septic encephalopathy

Next, we applied the NIR in vivo imaging to SE brain. To examine this, we studied whether DIC can be recorded with NIR imaging. **Figure 5** demonstrated lipopolysaccharide (LPS)-induced DIC. Eighteen hours after LPS, clots (arrowheads) can be recorded noninvasively (**Figure 5b**, middle). In the isolated brain, the number of clots remarkably increased in the SE brain (**Figure 6**). Conversely, the increased clots were similar to the control level in the presence of heparin (i.e., inhibitor of clots formation), suggesting that the NIR imaging can record DIC in SE brain.

What is the importance of these findings? In blood vessels of the brain, tissue factor activation including thrombin and fibrinogen which enhanced blood clot formation was occurred [114, 115], and this pathology finally led to multiple organ (e.g., lung, liver, kidney, and brain, etc.) dysfunction [116]. However, it has been difficult to visualize the pathological state of DIC because of a lack of an effective biomarker [117]. Our present findings developed a novel approach to analyze the pathological state of brain blood vessels in SE.

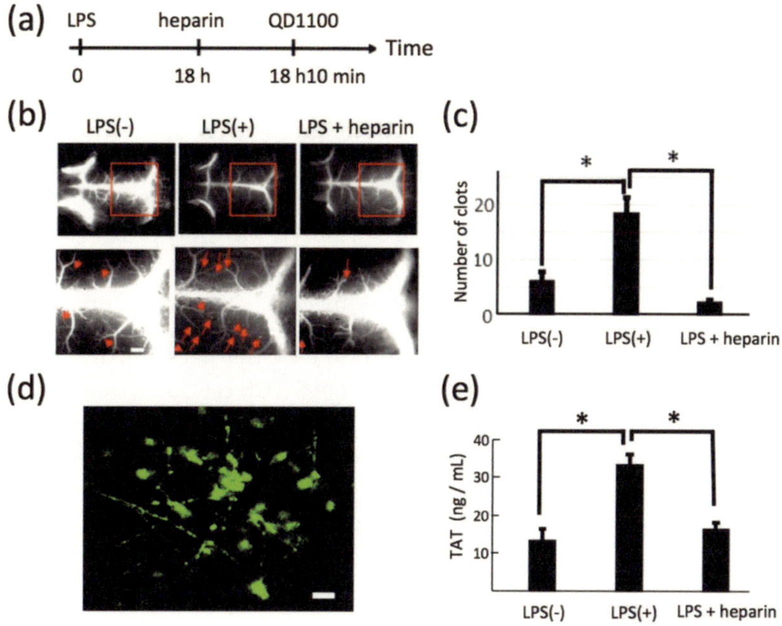

Figure 5. (a) Time course of experimental procedure for lipopolysaccharide (LPS) and heparin administration; (b) NIR fluorescence images (>1000 nm) of cerebral blood vessels before and after administration of LPS (LPS (−) and LPS (+)), and the image following additional administration of heparin (LPS + heparin) with scalp removed. Lower panel shows the magnification of the images shown by red rectangles. Arrowheads show clots. Scale bars: 1 mm; (c) statistical analyses of the clots in the cerebral vessels. *: $p < 0.05$, number of mice: LPS (−): $n = 5$, LPS (+): $n = 5$, LPS + heparin: $n = 3$; (d) immunofluorescence staining of LPS-treated cerebral blood vessels, where antifibrinogen antibody (Alexa Fluor 488) was used for staining of fibrinogen. Fibrinogen helps the formation of blood clots. Scale bar: 10 μm; (e) ELISA assays for thrombin–antithrombin complex (TAT) in blood plasma. *: $p < 0.05$, number of mice: LPS (−): $n = 5$, LPS (+): $n = 5$, LPS + heparin: $n = 3$. (Citation from Ref. [71]).

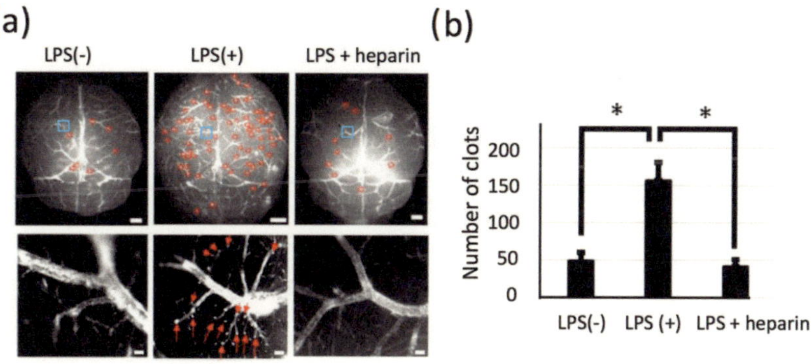

Figure 6. (a) Upper panel: NIR fluorescence images (>1000 nm) of cerebral blood vessels of isolated mouse brains. Left: LPS (−), Middle: LPS (+), Right: LPS + heparin. Red circles: clots. Blue squares: region of interests for the magnified views of lower panels. Scale bars: 1 mm. Lower panel: magnified NIR fluorescence image of cerebral blood vessels at the bregma. Red arrows: clots. Scale bars: 100 μm; (b) Number of clots for each mouse. *: $p < 0.05$, number of mice: LPS (−): $n = 5$, LPS (+): $n = 5$, LPS + heparin: $n = 4$. (Citation from Ref. [71]).

7. Future prospect

In this chapter, we introduce the application of NIR in vivo imaging to SE. Currently, imaging technology is confronted with a turning point. Although there are several noninvasive imaging technologies (PET, MRI, etc.), NIR noninvasive imaging can possibly record the faster time-dependent changes of pathological state in SE, though further developments of the imaging algorithm are required. In addition, the NIR imaging can label the distinct proteins by several specific antibodies and perform the multiple molecular in vivo imaging. Therefore, using the biomarker for SE, we may be able to visualize the novel pathophysiological mechanisms of SE.

Finally, in addition to our challenges, other candidate biomarkers which employ correlation to the pathological state of SE are recently addressed: S100β (i.e., astrocyte-secreting protein) [77, 118–120], free radicals [121, 122], ascorbate [123–125], and various neuropeptides [126]. In addition, adult neurogenesis was induced in a rat model of SE and the neurogenesis marker (e.g., 5-bromo-2′-deoxyuridine) might be useful [127]. In conclusion, these multidisciplinary approaches may overcome the pathophysiology and lead to innovative therapeutics for SE.

Acknowledgements

We thank Sumire Hino for secretary assistance, Dr. Jun Imamura for preparing **Figure 1**, Dr. Akitoshi Seiyama for critical reading of manuscript, and Kylius Wilkins for English corrections. This work is supported by Grant-in-Aid for Scientific Research of YI (24592734).

Author details

Yukio Imamura[1*], Yuki Murakami[2], Naoya Matsumoto[3], Hisatake Matsumoto[3], Satoko Mitani[4], Kentaro Shimizu[3], Hiroshi Ogura[3], Takeshi Shimazu[3] and Takashi Jin[1]

*Address all correspondence to: yukio.imamura@riken.jp

1 Laboratory for Nano-Bio Probes, Quantitative Biology Center, Riken, Japan

2 Laboratory of Developmental Neurobiology, Graduate School of Brain Science, Doshisha University, Japan

3 Department of Acute and Critical Care Center, Osaka University Hospital, Japan

4 Department of Nursing, School of Health Sciences, Gifu University of Medical Sciences, Gifu, Japan

References

[1] Imamura, Y., H. Wang, N. Matsumoto, T. Muroya, J. Shimazaki, H. Ogura, *et al.*, Interleukin-1beta causes long-term potentiation deficiency in a mouse model of septic encephalopathy. Neuroscience. 2011; **187**: 63-69.

[2] Rada, P., G.P. Mark, M.P. Vitek, R.M. Mangano, A.J. Blume, B. Beer, *et al.*, Interleukin-1 beta decreases acetylcholine measured by microdialysis in the hippocampus of freely moving rats. Brain Res. 1991; **550**(2): 287-290.

[3] Polito, A., F. Eischwald, A.L. Maho, A. Polito, E. Azabou, D. Annane, *et al.*, Pattern of brain injury in the acute setting of human septic shock. Crit Care. 2013; **17**(5): R204, DOI: 10.1186/cc12899.

[4] Gofton, T.E. and G.B. Young, Sepsis-associated encephalopathy. Nat Rev Neurol. 2012; **8**(10): 557-566.

[5] Streck, E.L., C.M. Comim, T. Barichello, and J. Quevedo, The septic brain. Neurochem Res. 2008; **33**: 2171-2177.

[6] Widmann, C.N. and M.T. Heneka, Long-term cerebral consequences of sepsis. Lancet Neurol. 2014; **13**(6): 630-636, DOI: 10.1016/s1474-4422(14)70017-1.

[7] Tsuruta, R. and Y. Oda, A clinical perspective of sepsis-associated delirium. J Intensive Care. 2016; **4**: 18, DOI: 10.1186/s40560-016-0145-4.

[8] Comim, C.M., L.C. Constantino, T. Barichello, E.L. Streck, J. Quevedo, and F. Dal-Pizzol, Cognitive impairment in the septic brain. Curr Neurovasc Res. 2009; **6**: 194-203.

[9] Luitse, M.J., C.J. van Asch, and C.J. Klijn, Deep coma and diffuse white matter abnormalities caused by sepsis-associated encephalopathy. Lancet. 2013; **381**(9884): 2222, DOI: 10.1016/s0140-6736(13)60682-0.

[10] Papadopoulos, M.C., D.C. Davies, R.F. Moss, D. Tighe, and E.D. Bennett, Pathophysiology of septic encephalopathy: a review. Crit Care Med. 2000; **28**: 3019-3024.

[11] Piva, S., V.A. McCreadie, and N. Latronico, Neuroinflammation in sepsis: sepsis associated delirium. Cardiovasc Hematol Disord Drug Targets. 2015; **15**(1): 10-18.

[12] Berisavac, II, V.V. Padjen, M.D. Ercegovac, G. Beslac-Bumbasirevic Lj, P. Stanarcevic, M.S. Stefanovic-Budimkic, *et al.*, Focal epileptic seizures, electroencephalography and outcome of sepsis associated encephalopathy-A pilot study. Clin Neurol Neurosurg. 2016; **148**: 60-66, DOI: 10.1016/j.clineuro.2016.06.013.

[13] Siami, S., D. Annane, and T. Sharshar, The encephalopathy in sepsis. Crit Care Clin. 2008; **24**(1): 67-82, viii, DOI: 10.1016/j.ccc.2007.10.001.

[14] Yamaguchi, H., T. Tanaka, A. Maruyama, and H. Nagase, Septic encephalopathy characterized by acute encephalopathy with biphasic seizures and late reduced diffusion and early nonconvulsive status epilepticus. Case Rep Neurol Med. 2016; **2016**: Article ID 7528238, DOI: 10.1155/2016/7528238.

[15] Young, G.B., C.F. Bolton, T.W. Austin, Y.M. Archibald, J. Gonder, and G.A. Wells, The encephalopathy associated with septic illness. Clin Invest Med. 1990; **13**: 297-304.

[16] Ziaja, M., Septic encephalopathy. Curr Neurol Neurosci Rep. 2013; **13**(10): 383, DOI: 10.1007/s11910-013-0383-y.

[17] Kafa, I.M., I. Ari, and M.A. Kurt, The peri-microvascular edema in hippocampal CA1 area in a rat model of sepsis. Neuropathology. 2007; **27**: 213-220.

[18] Kondo, A., C. Sugiura, Y. Fujii, T. Inoue, Y. Maegaki, and K. Ohno, Fulminant sepsis-associated encephalopathy in two children: serial neuroimaging findings and clinical course. Neuropediatrics. 2009; **40**(4): 157-161, DOI: 10.1055/s-0029-1243626.

[19] Sari, A., S. Yamashita, S. Ohosita, H. Ogasahara, K. Yamada, A. Yonei, *et al.*, Cerebrovascular reactivity to CO_2 in patients with hepatic or septic encephalopathy. Resuscitation. 1990; **19**(2): 125-134.

[20] Sweis, R., J. Ortiz, and J. Biller, Neurology of Sepsis. Curr Neurol Neurosci Rep. 2016; **16**(3): 21, DOI: 10.1007/s11910-016-0623-z.

[21] Lamar, C.D., R.A. Hurley, and K.H. Taber, Sepsis-associated encephalopathy: review of the neuropsychiatric manifestations and cognitive outcome. J Neuropsychiatr Clin Neurosci. 2011; **23**(3): 237-241, DOI: 10.1176/appi.neuropsych.23.3.23710.1176/jnp.23.3.jnp237.

[22] Gustot, T., F. Durand, D. Lebrec, J.L. Vincent, and R. Moreau, Severe sepsis in cirrhosis. Hepatology. 2009; **50**: 2022-2033.

[23] Rolando, N., J. Wade, M. Davalos, J. Wendon, J. Philpott-Howard, and R. Williams, The systemic inflammatory response syndrome in acute liver failure. Hepatology. 2000; **32**(4 Pt 1): 734-739, DOI: 10.1053/jhep.2000.17687.

[24] Tsai, M.H., Y.S. Peng, Y.C. Chen, N.J. Liu, Y.P. Ho, J.T. Fang, *et al.*, Adrenal insufficiency in patients with cirrhosis, severe sepsis and septic shock. Hepatology. 2006; **43**(4): 673-681, DOI: 10.1002/hep.21101.

[25] Wijdicks, E.F. and M. Stevens, The role of hypotension in septic encephalopathy following surgical procedures. Arch Neurol. 1992; **49**(6): 653-656.

[26] Berg, R.M., S. Taudorf, D.M. Bailey, C. Lundby, F.S. Larsen, B.K. Pedersen, *et al.*, Effects of lipopolysaccharide infusion on arterial levels and transcerebral exchange kinetics of glutamate and glycine in healthy humans. Apmis. 2012; **120**(9): 761-766, DOI: 10.1111/j.1600-0463.2012.02904.x.

[27] Ari, I., I.M. Kafa, and M.A. Kurt, Perimicrovascular edema in the frontal cortex in a rat model of intraperitoneal sepsis. Exp Neurol. 2006; **198**: 242-249.

[28] Papadopoulos, M.C., F.J. Lamb, R.F. Moss, D.C. Davies, D. Tighe, and E.D. Bennett, Faecal peritonitis causes oedema and neuronal injury in pig cerebral cortex. Clin Sci. (Lond). 1999; **96**: 461-466.

[29] Imamura, Y., N. Yoshikawa, Y. Murkami, S. Mitani, N. Matsumoto, H. Matsumoto, *et al.*, Effect of histone acetylation on N-methyl-D-aspartate 2B receptor subunits and interleukin-1 receptors in association with nociception-related somatosensory cortex dysfunction in a mouse model of sepsis. Shock. 2016; **45**(6): 660-667, DOI: 10.1097/SHK.0000000000000547.

[30] Wang, H., Y. Imamura, N. Matsumoto, N. Yoshikawa, J. Nakagawa, K. Yamakawa, *et al.*, Matrix metalloproteinase-9 triggers the gap junction impairment and somatosensory neuronal dysfunction in septic encephalopathy. Biochem Pharmacol: Open Access. 2013; **02**(01): 7, DOI: 10.4172/2167-0501.1000108.

[31] Anderson, S.T., S. Commins, P.N. Moynagh, and A.N. Coogan, Lipopolysaccharide-induced sepsis induces long-lasting affective changes in the mouse. Brain Behav Immun. 2015; **43**: 98-109, DOI: 10.1016/j.bbi.2014.07.007.

[32] Calsavara, A.C., D.H. Rodrigues, A.S. Miranda, P.A. Costa, C.X. Lima, M.C. Vilela, *et al.*, Late anxiety-like behavior and neuroinflammation in mice subjected to sublethal polymicrobial sepsis. Neurotox Res. 2013; **24**(2): 103-108, DOI: 10.1007/s12640-012-9364-1.

[33] Michels, M., A.S. Vieira, F. Vuolo, H.G. Zapelini, B. Mendonca, F. Mina, *et al.*, The role of microglia activation in the development of sepsis-induced long-term cognitive impairment. Brain Behav Immun. 2015; **43**: 54-59, DOI: 10.1016/j.bbi.2014.07.002.

[34] Gupta, R., S. Saigal, R. Joshi, P. Tagore, N. Rai, and K. Prasad, Unrecognized catatonia as a cause for delayed weaning in Intensive Care Unit. Indian J Crit Care Med. 2015; **19**(11): 693-694, DOI: 10.4103/0972-5229.169360.

[35] Imamura, Y., S. Hori, N. Matsumoto, K. Yamakawa, J. Nakagawa, J. Shimazaki, *et al.*, Septic encephalopathy. Encephalitis, Encephalomyelitis and Encephalopathies. Vol. 8. 2013: Nova Science Publisher. 163-176.

[36] Imamura, Y., H. Wang, N. Matsumoto, H. Ogura, T. Shimazu, T. Jin, *et al.*, Neurochemistry in the pathophysiology of septic encephalopathy. Neuroscience-Dealing with Frontiers ed. Neurochemistry, ed. M. Contreras. 2012, Croatias: In-tech Open Access Publisher.

[37] Basler, T., A. Meier-Hellmann, D. Bredle, and K. Reinhart, Amino acid imbalance early in septic encephalopathy. Intensive Care Med. 2002; **28**: 293-298.

[38] Berg, R.M., S. Taudorf, D.M. Bailey, C. Lundby, F.S. Larsen, B.K. Pedersen, *et al.*, Cerebral net exchange of large neutral amino acids after lipopolysaccharide infusion in healthy humans. Crit Care. 2010; **14**(1): R16, DOI: 10.1186/cc8873.

[39] Freund, H., S. Atamian, J. Holroyde, and J.E. Fischer, Plasma amino acids as predictors of the severity and outcome of sepsis. Ann Surg. 1979; **190**: 571-576.

[40] Nakamura, T., Y. Kawagoe, T. Matsuda, I. Ebihara, and H. Koide, Effects of polymyxin B-immobilized fiber hemoperfusion on amino acid imbalance in septic encephalopathy. Blood Purif. 2003; **21**: 282-286.

[41] Takezawa, J., N. Taenaka, M.K. Nishijima, T. Hirata, T. Okada, Y. Shimada, *et al.*, Amino acids and thiobarbituric acid reactive substances in cerebrospinal fluid and plasma of patients with septic encephalopathy. Crit Care Med. 1983; **11**(11): 876-879.

[42] Freund, H.R., M. Muggia-Sullam, R. LaFrance, J. Holroyde, and J.E. Fischer, Regional brain amino acid and neurotransmitter derangements during abdominal sepsis and

septic encephalopathy in the rat. The effect of amino acid infusions. Arch Surg. 1986; **121**: 209-216.

[43] Gao, R., M.Q. Kan, S.G. Wang, R.H. Yang, and S.G. Zhang, Disrupted tryptophan metabolism induced cognitive impairment in a mouse model of sepsis-associated encephalopathy. Inflammation. 2016; **39**(2): 550-560, DOI: 10.1007/s10753-015-0279-x.

[44] Sprung, C.L., F.B. Cerra, H.R. Freund, R.M. Schein, F.N. Konstantinides, E.H. Marcial, *et al.*, Amino acid alterations and encephalopathy in the sepsis syndrome. Crit Care Med. 1991; **19**: 753-757.

[45] Nishioku, T., S. Dohgu, F. Takata, T. Eto, N. Ishikawa, K.B. Kodama, *et al.*, Detachment of brain pericytes from the basal lamina is involved in disruption of the blood-brain barrier caused by lipopolysaccharide-induced sepsis in mice. Cell Mol Neurobiol. 2009; **29**: 309-316.

[46] Pytel, P. and J.J. Alexander, Pathogenesis of septic encephalopathy. Curr Opin Neurol. 2009; **22**: 283-287.

[47] Ballabh, P., A. Braun, and M. Nedergaard, The blood-brain barrier: an overview: structure, regulation, and clinical implications. Neurobiol Dis. 2004; **16**: 1-13.

[48] Varatharaj, A. and I. Galea, The blood-brain barrier in systemic inflammation. Brain Behav Immun. 2016; **60**: 1-12. DOI: 10.1016/j.bbi.2016.03.010.

[49] Nico, B. and D. Ribatti, Morphofunctional aspects of the blood-brain barrier. Curr Drug Metab. 2012; **13**: 50-60.

[50] Zhang, L.N., X.H. Wang, L. Wu, L. Huang, C.G. Zhao, Q.Y. Peng, *et al.*, Diagnostic and predictive levels of calcium-binding protein A8 and tumor necrosis factor receptor-associated factor 6 in sepsis-associated encephalopathy: a prospective observational study. Chin Med J (Engl). 2016; **129**(14): 1674-1681, DOI: 10.4103/0366-6999.185860.

[51] Berg, R.M., K. Moller, and D.M. Bailey, Neuro-oxidative-nitrosative stress in sepsis. J Cereb Blood Flow Metab. 2011; **31**(7): 1532-1544, DOI: 10.1038/jcbfm.2011.48.

[52] Bozza, F.A., J.C. D'Avila, C. Ritter, R. Sonneville, T. Sharshar, and F. Dal-Pizzol, Bioenergetics, mitochondrial dysfunction, and oxidative stress in the pathophysiology of septic encephalopathy. Shock. 2013; **39**(Suppl 1): 10-16, DOI: 10.1097/SHK.0b013e31828fade1.

[53] Hara, N., M. Chijiiwa, M. Yara, Y. Ishida, Y. Ogiwara, M. Inazu, *et al.*, Metabolomic analyses of brain tissue in sepsis induced by cecal ligation reveal specific redox alterations--protective effects of the oxygen radical scavenger edaravone. Shock. 2015; **44**(6): 578-584, DOI: 10.1097/shk.0000000000000465.

[54] Michels, M., L.G. Danielski, F. Dal-Pizzol, and F. Petronilho, Neuroinflammation: microglial activation during sepsis. Curr Neurovasc Res. 2014; **11**(3): 262-270.

[55] Wu, J., M. Zhang, S. Hao, M. Jia, M. Ji, L. Qiu, *et al.*, Mitochondria-targeted peptide reverses mitochondrial dysfunction and cognitive deficits in sepsis-associated encephalopathy. Mol Neurobiol. 2015; **52**(1): 783-791, DOI: 10.1007/s12035-014-8918-z.

[56] Handa, O., J. Stephen, and G. Cepinskas, Role of endothelial nitric oxide synthase-derived nitric oxide in activation and dysfunction of cerebrovascular endothelial cells during early onsets of sepsis. Am J Physiol Heart Circ Physiol. 2008; **295**(4): H1712-H1719, DOI: 10.1152/ajpheart.00476.2008.

[57] Zhou, T., L. Zhao, R. Zhan, Q. He, Y. Tong, X. Tian, *et al.*, Blood-brain barrier dysfunction in mice induced by lipopolysaccharide is attenuated by dapsone. Biochem Biophys Res Commun. 2014; **453**(3): 419-424, DOI: 10.1016/j.bbrc.2014.09.093.

[58] Pierrakos, C., A. Antoine, D. Velissaris, I. Michaux, P. Bulpa, P. Evrard, *et al.*, Transcranial doppler assessment of cerebral perfusion in critically ill septic patients: a pilot study. Ann Intensive Care. 2013; **3**: 28, DOI: 10.1186/2110-5820-3-28.

[59] Szatmari, S., T. Vegh, A. Csomos, J. Hallay, I. Takacs, C. Molnar, *et al.*, Impaired cerebrovascular reactivity in sepsis-associated encephalopathy studied by acetazolamide test. Crit Care. 2010; **14**: R50.

[60] Naito, Y., K. Yoshioka, K. Tanaka, K. Tatsumi, S. Kimura, and Y. Kasuya, Endothelin B receptor-mediated encephalopathic events in mouse sepsis model. Life Sci. 2014; **118**(2): 340-346, DOI: 10.1016/j.lfs.2014.03.012.

[61] Shimojo, N., S. Jesmin, S. Zaedi, S. Maeda, S. Gando, I. Yamaguchi, *et al.*, Alterations of gene expressions of preproET-1 and ET receptors in brains of endotoxemic Sprague-Dawley rats. Exp Biol Med. (Maywood). 2006; **231**: 1058-1063.

[62] Frister, A., C. Schmidt, N. Schneble, M. Brodhun, F.A. Gonnert, M. Bauer, *et al.*, Phosphoinositide 3-kinase gamma affects LPS-induced disturbance of blood-brain barrier via lipid kinase-independent control of cAMP in microglial cells. Neuromolecular Med. 2014; **16**(4): 704-713, DOI: 10.1007/s12017-014-8320-z.

[63] Pierrakos, C., R. Attou, L. Decorte, A. Kolyviras, S. Malinverni, P. Gottignies, *et al.*, Transcranial Doppler to assess sepsis-associated encephalopathy in critically ill patients. BMC Anesthesiol. 2014; **14**: 45, DOI: 10.1186/1471-2253-14-45.

[64] Ji, M.H., L.L. Qiu, H. Tang, L.S. Ju, X.R. Sun, H. Zhang, *et al.*, Sepsis-induced selective parvalbumin interneuron phenotype loss and cognitive impairments may be mediated by NADPH oxidase 2 activation in mice. J Neuroinflammat. 2015; **12**: 182, DOI: 10.1186/s12974-015-0401-x.

[65] Alexander, J.J., A. Jacob, P. Cunningham, L. Hensley, and R.J. Quigg, TNF is a key mediator of septic encephalopathy acting through its receptor, TNF receptor-1. Neurochem Int. 2008; **52**: 447-456.

[66] Erbas, O. and D. Taskiran, Sepsis-induced changes in behavioral stereotypy in rats; involvement of tumor necrosis factor-alpha, oxidative stress, and dopamine turnover. J Surg Res. 2014; **186**(1): 262-268, DOI: 10.1016/j.jss.2013.08.001.

[67] Flierl, M.A., P.F. Stahel, D. Rittirsch, M. Huber-Lang, A.D. Niederbichler, L.M. Hoesel, *et al.*, Inhibition of complement C5a prevents breakdown of the blood-brain barrier and pituitary dysfunction in experimental sepsis. Crit Care. 2009; **13**: R12.

[68] Jacob, A., L.K. Hensley, B.D. Safratowich, R.J. Quigg, and J.J. Alexander, The role of the complement cascade in endotoxin-induced septic encephalopathy. Lab Invest. 2007; **87**: 1186-1194.

[69] Sui, D.M., Q. Xie, W.J. Yi, S. Gupta, X.Y. Yu, J.B. Li, *et al.*, Resveratrol protects against sepsis-associated encephalopathy and inhibits the NLRP3/IL-1beta axis in microglia. Mediators Inflamm. 2016; **2016**: 1045657 Article ID 1045657, DOI: 10.1155/2016/1045657.

[70] Fang, J., Y. Lian, K. Xie, S. Cai, and P. Wen, Epigenetic modulation of neuronal apoptosis and cognitive functions in sepsis-associated encephalopathy. Neurol Sci. 2014; **35**(2): 283-288, DOI: 10.1007/s10072-013-1508-4.

[71] Imamura, Y., S. Yamada, S. Tsuboi, Y. Nakane, Y. Tsukasaki, A. Komatsuzaki, *et al.*, Near-infrared emitting PbS quantum dots for in vivo fluorescence imaging of the thrombotic state in septic mouse brain. Molecules. 2016; **21**(8): 1080.

[72] Li, R., J. Tong, Y. Tan, S. Zhu, J. Yang, and M. Ji, Low molecular weight heparin prevents lipopolysaccharide induced-hippocampus-dependent cognitive impairments in mice. Int J Clin Exp Pathol. 2015; **8**(8): 8881-8891.

[73] Chen, Q., W. Yu, J. Shi, J. Shen, T. Gao, J. Zhang, *et al.*, Insulin alleviates the inflammatory response and oxidative stress injury in cerebral tissues in septic rats. J Inflamm (Lond). 2014; **11**: 18, DOI: 10.1186/1476-9255-11-18.

[74] Hernandes, M.S., J.C. D'Avila, S.C. Trevelin, P.A. Reis, E.R. Kinjo, L.R. Lopes, *et al.*, The role of Nox2-derived ROS in the development of cognitive impairment after sepsis. J Neuroinflammation. 2014; **11**: 36, DOI: 10.1186/1742-2094-11-36.

[75] Lin, H.C. and F.J. Wan, Hyperbaric oxygenation reduces overexpression of c-Fos and oxidative stress in the brain stem of experimental endotoxemic rats. Intensive Care Med. 2008; **34**: 1122-1132.

[76] Li, L., Q. Sun, Y. Li, Y. Yang, Y. Yang, T. Chang, *et al.*, Overexpression of SIRT1 induced by resveratrol and inhibitor of miR-204 suppresses activation and proliferation of microglia. J Mol Neurosci. 2015; **56**(4): 858-867. DOI: 10.1007/s12031-015-0526-5.

[77] Hamed, S.A., E.A. Hamed, and M.M. Abdella, Septic encephalopathy: relationship to serum and cerebrospinal fluid levels of adhesion molecules, lipid peroxides and S-100B protein. Neuropediatrics. 2009; **40**: 66-72.

[78] Liu, J., D. Zhao, C. Liu, T. Ding, L. Yang, X. Yin, *et al.*, Prion protein participates in the protection of mice from lipopolysaccharide infection by regulating the inflammatory process. J Mol Neurosci. 2015; **55**(1): 279-287, DOI: 10.1007/s12031-014-0319-2.

[79] Kondo, S., S. Kohsaka, and S. Okabe, Long-term changes of spine dynamics and microglia after transient peripheral immune response triggered by LPS in vivo. Mol Brain. 2011; **4**: 27.

[80] Freund, H.R., M. Muggia-Sullam, J. Peiser, and E. Melamed, Brain neurotransmitter profile is deranged during sepsis and septic encephalopathy in the rat. J Surg Res. 1985; **38**: 267-271.

[81] Davies, D.C., Blood-brain barrier breakdown in septic encephalopathy and brain tumours. J Anat. 2002; **200**: 639-646.

[82] Kadoi, Y., S. Saito, F. Kunimoto, T. Imai, and T. Fujita, Impairment of the brain beta-adrenergic system during experimental endotoxemia. J Surg Res. 1996; **61**: 496-502.

[83] Soejima, Y., Y. Fujii, T. Ishikawa, H. Takeshita, and T. Maekawa, Local cerebral glucose utilization in septic rats. Crit Care Med. 1990; **18**: 423-427.

[84] Dal-Pizzol, F., C.D. Tomasi, and C. Ritter, Septic encephalopathy: does inflammation drive the brain crazy? Rev Bras Psiquiatr. 2014; **36**(3): 251-258.

[85] Zhang, Q.H., Z.Y. Sheng, and Y.M. Yao, Septic encephalopathy: when cytokines interact with acetylcholine in the brain. Mil Med Res. 2014; **12**: 0, DOI: 10.1186/2054-9369-1-20.

[86] Zhu, S.Z., W.P. Huang, L.Q. Huang, Y.L. Han, Q.P. Han, G.F. Zhu, *et al.*, Huperzine A protects sepsis associated encephalopathy by promoting the deficient cholinergic nervous function. Neurosci Lett. 2016; **631**: 70-78, DOI: 10.1016/j.neulet.2016.07.009.

[87] Serantes, R., F. Arnalich, M. Figueroa, M. Salinas, E. Andres-Mateos, R. Codoceo, *et al.*, Interleukin-1beta enhances GABAA receptor cell-surface expression by a phosphatidylinositol 3-kinase/Akt pathway: relevance to sepsis-associated encephalopathy. J Biol Chem. 2006; **281**: 14632-14643.

[88] Taccone, F.S., S. Scolletta, F. Franchi, K. Donadello, and M. Oddo, Brain perfusion in sepsis. Curr Vasc Pharmacol. 2013; **11**(2): 170-186.

[89] Kafa, I.M., S. Bakirci, M. Uysal, and M.A. Kurt, Alterations in the brain electrical activity in a rat model of sepsis-associated encephalopathy. Brain Res. 2010; **1354**: 217-226.

[90] Zauner, C., A. Gendo, L. Kramer, G.C. Funk, E. Bauer, P. Schenk, *et al.*, Impaired subcortical and cortical sensory evoked potential pathways in septic patients. Crit Care Med. 2002; **30**: 1136-1139.

[91] Bolton, C.F., Electrophysiologic studies of critically ill patients. Muscle Nerve. 1987; **10**(2): 129-135, DOI: 10.1002/mus.880100205.

[92] Teener, J.W. and M.M. Rich, Dysregulation of sodium channel gating in critical illness myopathy. J Muscle Res Cell Motil. 2006; **27**: 291-296.

[93] Iacobone, E., J. Bailly-Salin, A. Polito, D. Friedman, R.D. Stevens, and T. Sharshar, Sepsis-associated encephalopathy and its differential diagnosis. Crit Care Med. 2009; **37**(10 Suppl): S331-S336, DOI: 10.1097/CCM.0b013e3181b6ed58.

[94] Oddo, M. and F.S. Taccone, How to monitor the brain in septic patients? Minerva Anestesiol. 2015; **81**(7): 776-788.

[95] Kaplan, P.W. and A.O. Rossetti, EEG patterns and imaging correlations in encephalopathy: encephalopathy part II. J Clin Neurophysiol. 2011; **28**(3): 233-251, DOI: 10.1097/WNP.0b013e31821c33a0.

[96] Young, G.B., C.F. Bolton, Y.M. Archibald, T.W. Austin, and G.A. Wells, The electroencephalogram in sepsis-associated encephalopathy. J Clin Neurophysiol. 1992; **9**: 145-152.

[97] Lin, L.C., Y.Y. Chen, W.T. Lee, H.L. Chen, and R.C. Yang, Heat shock pretreatment attenuates sepsis-associated encephalopathy in LPS-induced septic rats. Brain Dev. 2010; 32: 371-377.

[98] Bragatti, J.A., A.M. Mattos, H. Bastes, and R.S. Riesgo, Alpha coma pattern in a child. Clin EEG Neurosci. 2008; 39(4): 206-209.

[99] Hosokawa, K., N. Gaspard, F. Su, M. Oddo, J.L. Vincent, and F.S. Taccone, Clinical neurophysiological assessment of sepsis-associated brain dysfunction: a systematic review. Crit Care. 2014; **18**(6): 674, DOI: 10.1186/s13054-014-0674-y.

[100] Stubbs, D.J., A.K. Yamamoto, and D.K. Menon, Imaging in sepsis-associated encephalopathy[mdash]insights and opportunities. Nat Rev Neurol. 2013; 9(10): 551-561, DOI: 10.1038/nrneurol.2013.177.

[101] Sharshar, T., R. Carlier, F. Bernard, C. Guidoux, J.-P. Brouland, O. Nardi, et al., Brain lesions in septic shock: a magnetic resonance imaging study. Intensive Care Med. 2007; 33(5): 798-806, DOI: 10.1007/s00134-007-0598-y.

[102] Bozza, F.A., P. Garteiser, M.F. Oliveira, S. Doblas, R. Cranford, D. Saunders, et al., Sepsis-associated encephalopathy: a magnetic resonance imaging and spectroscopy study. J Cereb Blood Flow Metab. 2010; 30: 440-448.

[103] Finelli, P.F. and D.F. Uphoff, Magnetic resonance imaging abnormalities with septic encephalopathy. J Neurol Neurosurg Psychiatry. 2004; 75: 1189-1191.

[104] Gotz, T., A. Gunther, O.W. Witte, F.M. Brunkhorst, G. Seidel, and F. Hamzei, Long-term sequelae of severe sepsis: cognitive impairment and structural brain alterations - an MRI study (LossCog MRI). BMC Neurol. 2014; 14: 145, DOI: 10.1186/1471-2377-14-145.

[105] Semmler, A., S. Hermann, F. Mormann, M. Weberpals, S.A. Paxian, T. Okulla, et al., Sepsis causes neuroinflammation and concomitant decrease of cerebral metabolism. J Neuroinflammation. 2008; 5: 38.

[106] Weberpals, M., M. Hermes, S. Hermann, M.P. Kummer, D. Terwel, A. Semmler, et al., NOS2 gene deficiency protects from sepsis-induced long-term cognitive deficits. J Neurosci. 2009; 29: 14177-14184.

[107] Joo, C., H. Balci, Y. Ishitsuka, C. Buranachai, and T. Ha, Advances in single-molecule fluorescence methods for molecular biology. Annu Rev Biochem. 2008; 77: 51-76, DOI: 10.1146/annurev.biochem.77.070606.101543.

[108] Terai, T. and T. Nagano, Fluorescent probes for bioimaging applications. Curr Opin Chem Biol. 2008; 12(5): 515-521, DOI: 10.1016/j.cbpa.2008.08.007.

[109] Weissleder, R., A clearer vision for in vivo imaging. Nat Biotechnol. 2001; **19**(4): 316-317, DOI: 10.1038/86684.

[110] Jin, T. and Y. Imamura, Applications of highly bright PbS quantum dots to non-invasive near-infrared fluorescence imaging in the second optical window. ECS J Solid State Sci Technol. 2016; 5(1): R3138-R3145, DOI: 10.1149/2.0171601jss.

[111] Taccone, F.S., F. Su, C. Pierrakos, X. He, S. James, O. Dewitte, et al., Cerebral microcirculation is impaired during sepsis: an experimental study. Crit Care. 2010; 14: R140.

[112] Blauhut, B., H. Kramar, H. Vinazzer, and H. Bergmann, Substitution of antithrombin III in shock and DIC: a randomized study. Thromb Res. 1985; 39(1): 81-89.

[113] Iba, T., I. Nagaoka, and M. Boulat, The anticoagulant therapy for sepsis-associated disseminated intravascular coagulation. Thromb Res. 2013; 131(5): 383-389, DOI: 10.1016/j.thromres.2013.03.012.

[114] Semeraro, N., C.T. Ammollo, F. Semeraro, and M. Colucci, Sepsis-associated disseminated intravascular coagulation and thromboembolic disease. Mediterr J Hematol Infect Dis. 2010; 2(3): e2010024, DOI: 10.4084/MJHID.2010.024.

[115] ten Cate, H., S.H. Schoenmakers, R. Franco, J.J. Timmerman, A.P. Groot, C.A. Spek, et al., Microvascular coagulopathy and disseminated intravascular coagulation. Crit Care Med. 2001; 29(7 Suppl): S95-S97; discussion S97-98.

[116] Ziaja, M., Sepsis and septic encephalopathy: characteristics and experimental models. Folia Neuropathol. 2012; 50(3): 231-239.

[117] Zampieri, F.G., M. Park, F.S. Machado, and L.C. Azevedo, Sepsis-associated encephalopathy: not just delirium. Clinics (Sao Paulo). 2011; 66(10): 1825-1831.

[118] Panni, J.K. and M.K. Panni, Changes in S100B levels rather than absolute values may be a better marker of severity of septic encephalopathy. Br J Anaesth. 2008; 100(3): 419; author reply 419-420, DOI: 10.1093/bja/aen009.

[119] Piazza, O., E. Russo, S. Cotena, G. Esposito, and R. Tufano, Elevated S100B levels do not correlate with the severity of encephalopathy during sepsis. Br J Anaesth. 2007; 99(4): 518-521, DOI: 10.1093/bja/aem201.

[120] Spapen, H., D.N. Nguyen, J. Troubleyn, L. Huyghens, and J. Schiettecatte, Drotrecogin alfa (activated) may attenuate severe sepsis-associated encephalopathy in clinical septic shock. Crit Care. 2010; 14: R54.

[121] Towner, R.A., P. Garteiser, F. Bozza, N. Smith, D. Saunders, J.C. d' Avila, et al., In vivo detection of free radicals in mouse septic encephalopathy using molecular MRI and immuno-spin trapping. Free Radic Biol Med. 2013; 65: 828-837, DOI: 10.1016/j.freeradbiomed.2013.08.172.

[122] Yokoo, H., S. Chiba, K. Tomita, M. Takashina, H. Sagara, S. Yagisita, et al., Neurodegenerative evidence in mice brains with cecal ligation and puncture-induced sepsis: preventive effect of the free radical scavenger edaravone. PLoS One. 2012; **7**(12): e51539, DOI: 10.1371/journal.pone.0051539.

[123] Huang, Y.N., C.C. Lai, C.T. Chiu, J.J. Lin, and J.Y. Wang, L-ascorbate attenuates the endotoxin-induced production of inflammatory mediators by inhibiting MAPK activation and NF-kappaB translocation in cortical neurons/glia Cocultures. PLoS One. 2014; 9(7): e97276, DOI: 10.1371/journal.pone.0097276.

[124] Voigt, K., A. Kontush, H.J. Stuerenburg, D. Muench-Harrach, H.C. Hansen, and K. Kunze, Decreased plasma and cerebrospinal fluid ascorbate levels in patients with septic encephalopathy. Free Radic Res. 2002; 36: 735-739.

[125] Wilson, J.X. and F. Wu, Vitamin C in sepsis. Subcell Biochem. 2012; 56: 67-83, DOI: 10.1007/978-94-007-2199-9_5.

[126] Pinheiro da Silva, F., M.C. Machado, and I.T. Velasco, Neuropeptides in sepsis: from brain pathology to systemic inflammation. Peptides. 2013; 44: 135-138, DOI: 10.1016/j.peptides.2013.03.029.

[127] Bakirci, S., I.M. Kafa, M. Uysal, and M. Ayberk Kurt, Increased adult neurogenesis in the subventricular zone in a rat model of sepsis. Neurosci Lett. 2011; 497(1): 27-31, DOI: 10.1016/j.neulet.2011.04.014.